Maryland Campground Locator Map

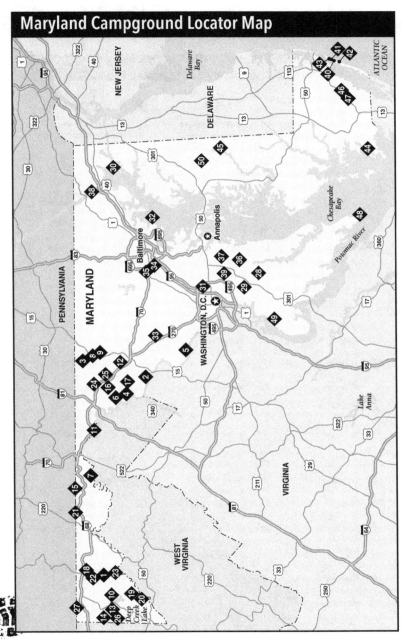

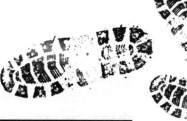

Maryland Campground Map Legend

	→	▲	🏕 🏕 🏕 ⌂ ⌂ ⌂ ⌂
North indicator	**Off-map or pinpoint-indication arrow**	**Campground name and location**	**Individual tent sites, RV sites, cabins, and cottages**

△ ⚠	Annapolis ✪	Baltimore ●	NATIONAL FOREST STATE PARK	🏇 ----- Main Trail
Group site	**Capital**	**City or town**	**Public lands**	**Hiking and equestrian trails**

⟨70⟩	⟨522⟩ ⟨40⟩ ⟨ALT 40⟩	⟨272⟩ ⟨4⟩	Bee Oak Rd
Interstate highways	**US highways**	**State roads**	**Other roads**

-----------	*Patuxent River*	*Deep Creek Lake*
Dirt/gravel roads	**River or stream**	**Lake or pond**

≍	Bridge or tunnel	🛝	Playground	⊼	Picnic area
♨	Amphitheater	🅿	Parking	🏠	Sheltered picnic area
🥛	Water access	🚤	Marina or boat ramp	♨	Dump station
♿	Wheelchair accessible	☎	Telephone	🔥	Fire pit
🚻	Restroom	🏊	Swimming	🎣	Fishing area
◑◐	Pit toilet	♞	Ranger station	◎	Range
🗑	Trash disposal	🛶	Canoe put-in	🚿	Showers
🛒	Store	⌐	Gazebo	🏊	Swimming area
🍴	Restaurant	▣	Laundry	$	Pay station
🏹	Archery range	🗼	Tree house	🥾	Guided trail
?	Information	▲	Peak	✚	First aid
⚑	Gate				

OVERVIEW-MAP KEY

:: OTHER TITLES IN THIS SERIES

Best Tent Camping: Arizona
Best Tent Camping: The Carolinas
Best Tent Camping: Colorado
Best Tent Camping: Florida
Best Tent Camping: Georgia
Best Tent Camping: Illinois
Best Tent Camping: Kentucky
Best Tent Camping: Michigan
Best Tent Camping: Minnesota
Best Tent Camping: Missouri and the Ozarks
Best Tent Camping: Montana
Best Tent Camping: New England
Best Tent Camping: New Jersey
Best Tent Camping: New Mexico
Best Tent Camping: New York State
Best Tent Camping: Northern California
Best Tent Camping: Ohio
Best Tent Camping: Oregon
Best Tent Camping: Pennsylvania
Best Tent Camping: The Southern Appalachian and Smoky Mountains
Best Tent Camping: Southern California
Best Tent Camping: Tennessee
Best Tent Camping: Texas
Best Tent Camping: Utah
Best Tent Camping: Virginia
Best Tent Camping: Washington
Best Tent Camping: West Virginia
Best Tent Camping: Wisconsin

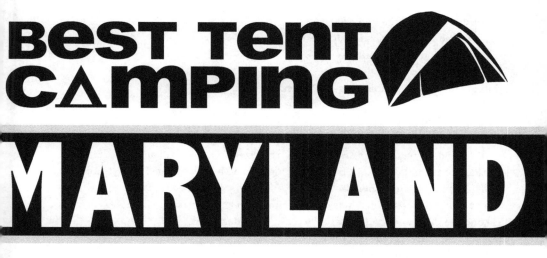

BEST TENT CAMPING
MARYLAND

**YOUR CAR-CAMPING GUIDE TO SCENIC BEAUTY,
THE SOUNDS OF NATURE,
AND AN ESCAPE FROM CIVILIZATION**

2nd Edition

EVAN BALKAN

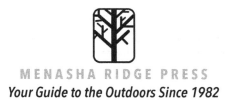

MENASHA RIDGE PRESS
Your Guide to the Outdoors Since 1982

Best Tent Camping: Maryland, 2nd Edition

Published by Menasha Ridge Press
Distributed by Publishers Group West
Second edition, first printing

Library of Congress Cataloging-in-Publication Data

Names: Balkan, Evan, 1972-
Title: Best tent camping, Maryland : your car-camping guide to scenic beauty,
    the sounds of nature, and an escape from civilization / Evan Balkan.
Description: 2nd Edition. | Birmingham, Alabama : Menasha Ridge Press, [2016] |
    "Distributed by Publishers Group West"—T.p. verso. | First edition title:
    The best in tent camping, Maryland : a guide for car campers who hate RVs,
    concrete slabs, and loud portable stereos. | Includes index.
Identifiers: LCCN 2015043561 (print) | LCCN 2015045297 (ebook) |
    ISBN 9780897324151 (pbk.) | ISBN 9780897324199 (eBook) |
    ISBN 9781634041881 (hardcover)
Subjects: LCSH: Camp sites, facilities, etc.—Maryland—Directories. |
    Camping—Maryland—Guidebooks. | Maryland—Guidebooks.
Classification: LCC GV191.42.M3 B35 2016 (print) | LCC GV191.42.M3 (ebook) |
    DDC 796.5409752—dc23
LC record available at http://lccn.loc.gov/2015043561

Cover design by Scott McGrew
Cover photo © Patrick Davis / Alamy Stock Photo; interior photos by Evan Balkan
Text design by Annie Long
Cartography by Steve Jones and Evan Balkan
Indexing by Rich Carlson

Menasha Ridge Press
    An imprint of AdventureKEEN
    2204 First Ave. S., Suite 102
    Birmingham, AL 35233
    menasharidgepress.com

Visit **menasharidge.com** for a complete listing of our books and for ordering information. Contact us at our website, at **facebook.com/menasharidge**, at **twitter.com/menasharidge**, or at **blog.menasharidge .com** with questions or comments.

CONTENTS

BEST CAMPGROUNDS

PREFACE

I've had the good fortune to travel quite a bit, visiting some 25 countries on four continents and more than 30 American states. When I travel, comparisons to home are inevitable. Maryland, by most accounts, should come up short. After all, while Maryland enjoys a rich history (I grew up just a mile from a church built in the late 1600s), what is it against Machu Picchu, the Roman Coliseum, or the pyramids at Giza? Maryland's high point tops out at just over 3,300 feet—what's that against major peaks in the Rockies, the Andes, or the Himalayas? Yes, I've spent many happy hours frolicking in the green, pounding surf of the mid-Atlantic off Ocean City, but can it compare to the crystal clarity of Lake Tahoe or the stupendous natural splendor of the Pacific off California's Big Sur?

Believe it or not, I find that, invariably, my little Maryland manages to hold its own, thank you very much.

Perhaps an objective judge would find my favorable comparisons ridiculous, and I'll concede that there's something of a hometown bias going on, but I make my complimentary judgments without embarrassment. In fact, when I first visited Lake Tahoe and California's Pacific Coast, for example, it was October, and while virtually everything I saw in beautiful northern California was brown and scrubby, my flight home gave me one more reminder why I love Maryland so much. During the airplane's descent, I watched with joy as we glided over the spiraling kaleidoscope of color that is autumn in Maryland.

I once read that when you take into account all of Maryland's tributaries, the state actually has more miles of shoreline than California. I find that claim dubious, though I suppose some favorable formulation will allow one to arrive at that conclusion. Of course, there are so many competing claims for superlatives—for instance, I've seen no fewer than three locales boasting that they are the world's most isolated, populated spots—it seems that the veracity of claims of highest, deepest, wettest, oldest, and so on has to be measured against formulation and whatever particular tourist board is making the assertion. Nevertheless, it is indisputable that if you take the Chesapeake Bay, the Atlantic Ocean, and all the tributaries in the Bay watershed, you could spend a lifetime paddling the shores of all of them. Still, for my money, plunk me down in the mountains, and I'm content. Maryland's west is full of great recreational activities, and the camping is no exception. Even in the crowded central corridor between Baltimore and Washington, D.C., camping and other recreational opportunities abound.

In short, Marylanders enjoy something of an embarrassment of riches when it comes to the great outdoors. So get out there and enjoy it.

—Evan Balkan

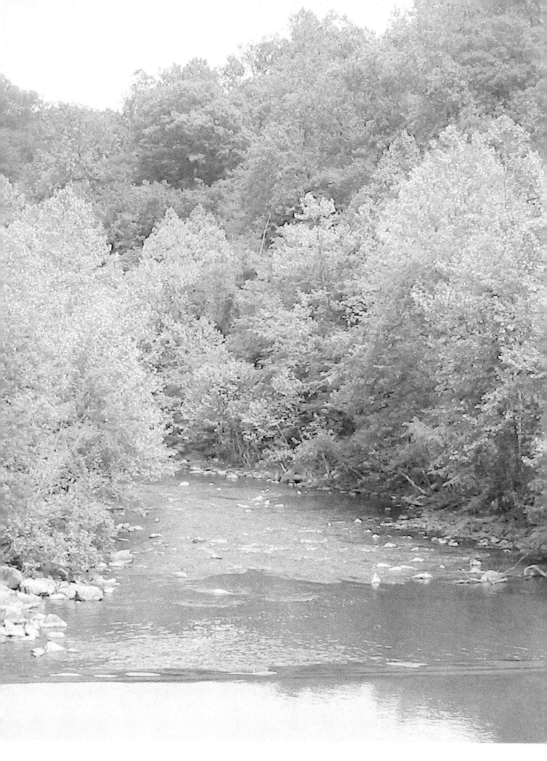

The Hilton Area of Patapsco Valley State Park (see page 126)

INTRODUCTION

How to Use This Guidebook

We at **Menasha Ridge Press** welcome you to *Best Tent Camping: Maryland.* Whether you're new to this activity or you've been sleeping in your portable outdoor shelter over decades of outdoor adventures, please review the following information. It explains how we have worked with the author to organize this book and how you can make the best use of it.

:: THE RATINGS & RATING CATEGORIES

As with all of the books in the publisher's *Best Tent Camping* series, this guidebook's author personally experienced dozens of campgrounds and campsites to select the top 50 locations in this region. Within that universe of 50 sites, each was then ranked in the six categories described below. Each campground in this guidebook is superlative in its own way. For example, a site may be rated only one star in one category but perhaps five stars in another category. This rating system allows you to choose your destination based on the attributes that are most important to you. Though these ratings are subjective, they're still excellent guidelines for finding the perfect camping experience for you and your companions.

Evaluating campgrounds requires some finesse, and in the end it is more of an art than a science. For a quick summary of what qualities make these campgrounds worth visiting, each is rated on six attributes: beauty, privacy, spaciousness, quiet, security, and cleanliness. A five-star scale is used. Not every campground in this book can pull a high score in every category. Sometimes a very worthwhile campground is located on terrain that makes it difficult to provide a lot of space, for example. In these cases, look for high marks in beauty or quiet to trump room to stretch out. In every case, the star rating system is a handy tool to help you pinpoint the campground that will fit your personal requirements.

★ ★ ★ ★ ★   The site is **ideal** in that category.

★ ★ ★ ★   The site is **exemplary** in that category.

★ ★ ★   The site is **very good** in that category.

★ ★   The site is **above average** in that category.

★   The site is **acceptable** in that category.

Beauty

This category includes the area that extends beyond the campground itself. Easy access to thick forest, clear streams, or stupendous views gives a campground a high ranking, regardless of whether the specific sites themselves are apt to awe you.

Privacy

This category refers to the ease with which campers in the next site can hear you and vice versa. Few campgrounds in this book don't offer at least a small green buffer between sites, but the ranking in this category will give you a good idea of how much.

Spaciousness

Spaciousness refers to the physical dimensions of the campsites. If you are in a group, for example, this may be a top concern.

Quiet

This is a difficult category to measure because different times of the year, times of the week, and luck of the neighborly draw will determine your experience. However, every effort was made to talk with other campers, rangers, and park employees at each campground to try to get a fair sense of what visitors can expect any time of the year.

Security

DNR-run campgrounds are invariably safe. Almost all have a camp host and easy access to ranger offices. Park police regularly patrol state campgrounds as well. Some of the more remote campgrounds received a lower rating for safety simply because there might be no one around to deter crime, so you might be more vulnerable. Of course, this isolation is what attracts many people to these places. In general, Maryland campgrounds are very safe and secure.

Cleanliness

This is self-explanatory but refers to the amount of litter you might find at the campground. Overflowing trash cans and restrooms that didn't look well maintained were cause for knocking off a few stars in this category.

:: THE CAMPGROUND PROFILE

Each profile contains a concise but informative narrative of the campground and individual sites. Not only is the property described, but readers can also get a general idea of the recreational opportunities available in the area and perhaps suggestions for touristy activities. This descriptive text is enhanced with three helpful sidebars: Ratings, Key Information, and Getting There (accurate driving directions that lead you to the campground from the nearest major roadway, along with GPS coordinates).

:: THE OVERVIEW MAP, MAP KEY, AND LEGEND

Use the overview map on the inside front cover to assess the exact location of each campground. The campground's number appears not only on the overview map but also on the map key facing the overview map, in the table of contents, and on the profile's first page. This book is organized by region, as indicated in the table of contents.

A map legend that details the symbols found on the campground-layout maps appears on the inside back cover.

:: CAMPGROUND-LAYOUT MAPS

Each profile includes a detailed map of campground sites, internal roads, facilities, and other key items.

:: GPS CAMPGROUND-ENTRANCE COORDINATES

Readers can easily access all campgrounds in this book by using the directions given and the overview map, which shows at least one major road leading into the area. But for those who enjoy using GPS technology to navigate, the book includes coordinates for each campground's entrance in latitude and longitude, expressed in degrees, minutes, and seconds. For more on GPS technology, visit **usgs.gov.**

A note of caution: Actual GPS devices will easily guide you to any of these campgrounds, but users of smartphone mapping apps will find that cell phone service is often unavailable in the hills and hollows where many of these hideaways are located.

About This Book

M**any Marylanders** like to boast about the state's unofficial nickname, "America in Miniature." Bestowed on the state by National Geographic founding editor Gilbert Grosvenor, it's not a hyperbolic moniker. For a relatively small state—the country's ninth smallest in area (with number ten almost twice the size)—Maryland packs in a tremendous amount of physical diversity. Having both mountains and ocean shoreline in the same state is a real plus; however, many states on the East Coast can make the same claim. What sets Maryland apart from these is the presence of Chesapeake Bay, the country's largest estuary. The Bay's central and massive presence in Maryland means its effects are far-reaching; in addition to being a major source of recreation, the Bay's bounty formed a major part of the state's economy from Maryland's founding in the 17th century through the next three centuries.

Generally, the state is carved by three distinct fault lines, which run geographically as well as politically and culturally. Western Maryland is mountainous and retains some vestiges of its status as part of America's first frontier—the Alleghany range of the Appalachians, the first natural barrier to European immigrants heading west. Central Maryland is urban and suburban, anchored by Baltimore in the north and Washington, D.C., in the south. The corridor between these two major cities is home to high-end service industries and a plethora of research institutions, as well as pleasant residential zones. Large swaths of the natural world are surprisingly abundant and—not surprisingly—cherished. Then there is southern Maryland and the Eastern Shore, both dominated by water. Mostly this means the Chesapeake Bay and its tributaries, but there's also the Atlantic Ocean, forming Maryland's eastern boundary.

Accordingly, I've separated the camping locations in this book by these distinct zones listed above. Virtually any Maryland resident can reach at least a few of the camping destinations in this book in a quick trip, certainly in less than an hour. Most of the state's population is clustered in the central, urban zone. We can reach all of the book's destinations in less than four hours, and many, if not most, in less than three or even two.

In choosing which campgrounds to include, I tried hard to keep in mind the "typical" camper, meaning in this case an amalgam of all the campers I met while doing research for the two editions of this book. My personal preference is for out-of-the-way spots where one has to be fully self-sufficient, places where you can blissfully lose all the trappings of modernity for a few days. My bias for such places most probably comes through in my descriptions of the camping destinations, such as the primitive sites in the state forests at Green Ridge, Potomac, and Garrett. However, I am aware that many more campers like easy access to facilities and don't want to travel too far or with too many jugs of potable water. Thus, I included many campgrounds that offer anything a camper could want. For instance, new to this edition is Watkins Regional Park in Prince George's County, which fits that description. However, I was careful to exclude campgrounds that were overrun with RVs and where finding silence and privacy were virtual impossibilities. Don't misunderstand: I've shared campground space with RVers and still enjoyed the experience immensely. Thus, a campground with a lot of RVs wasn't automatically excluded from this book. Besides, more and more campgrounds are geared toward catering to the RV set. But rest assured, you'll find many campgrounds in this book that are impossible for RV owners to reach or where RVs aren't even allowed. Also new to the 2nd edition are the campsites along the Patuxent Water Trail; there are certainly no RVs there.

:: WEATHER

Continuing on the "Maryland-has-it-all" theme, the state offers four very distinct seasons—though, as any denizen knows, nothing is absolute. For example, the winter of 2013–2014 was unusually cold, windy, and snowy (and felt relentless, frankly), and the following summer was mild and simply lovely, a break from the usual crush of Maryland's humid middle months. Winter can range from mild to downright frigid. The western part of the state is known for heavy snowfalls. Far western Garrett County, home to quite a few campgrounds in this book, actually sits west of the Eastern Continental Divide and sees, on average, some 140 inches of snow per season and routinely surpasses 200 inches. Generally speaking, spring is lovely—cold to start but yielding to gradually warmer temperatures and lengthening days. Forests burst into color and migratory songbirds make their return. Summer can be a bear, with high temperatures and crushing humidity, but the long days and sense of freedom attendant summer everywhere more than make up for that. Fall is sublime. For my money, it's the best of all seasons. The fall foliage explodes. (Head out to Western Maryland, especially, for this, as few places anywhere rival the shows in the western forests; in fact, in 2014, *Travel + Leisure* magazine named Garrett County's Oakland the best town in the country for seeing fall foliage. Who says you need to head to New England?) Fall usually sees a steady string of gorgeous days and cool nights, with plenty of sun and warmth to get you out there amid the colors, with leaves tenaciously hanging on well into November. In my opinion, this is the best time to camp in Maryland.

:: FIRST AID KIT

A useful first aid kit may contain more items than you might think necessary. These are just the basics. Prepackaged kits in waterproof bags (Atwater Carey and Adventure Medical make them) are available. As a preventive measure, take along sunscreen and insect repellent. Even though quite a few items are listed here, they pack down into a small space:

- Ace bandages or Spenco joint wraps
- Adhesive bandages, such as Band-Aids
- Antibiotic ointment (Neosporin or the generic equivalent)
- Antiseptic or disinfectant, such as Betadine or hydrogen peroxide
- Aspirin or acetaminophen
- Benadryl or the generic equivalent, diphenhydramine (in case of allergic reactions)
- Butterfly-closure bandages
- Epinephrine in a prefilled syringe (for people known to have severe allergic reactions)
- Gauze (one roll and six 4- x 4-inch compress pads)
- LED flashlight or headlamp
- Matches or pocket lighter
- Moist towelettes
- Moleskin/Spenco 2nd Skin
- Pocketknife or multipurpose tool
- Waterproof first aid tape
- Whistle (more effective in signaling rescuers than your voice)

:: ANIMAL AND PLANT HAZARDS
Snakes

The prospect of being bitten by a snake should never deter a camper in Maryland. The state has only two native poisonous snakes: northern copperheads, which you may see, usually near water, in central, southern, and eastern Maryland; and timber rattlers, which live in the mountainous, western part of the state. Although the chances of being bitten by a snake are slim, take proper caution. For good information on snakes in Maryland, visit **dnr.state .md.us/wildlife/vsnakes.asp.**

Ticks

All outdoor recreationists in Maryland should be concerned about ticks. Your best protection is to be vigilant: Check yourself frequently and look closely. Often, the smaller the tick, the greater the chance for subsequent serious health problems. Tiny deer ticks (black-legged ticks), for example, carry Lyme disease; if you see a bull's-eye rash radiating from a tender red spot, see a doctor right away. If you experience flulike symptoms (intense malaise, fever, chills, and a headache) a day or two after camping, look very hard for the telltale bull's-eye rash and see a doctor to alleviate any concerns. If you find a tick attached to your skin, gently remove it with tweezers, taking care to pull it off gently so the mouthpart does not break off and remain attached. In general, ticks pose a major threat only during the warmest months of summer, but an unseasonably mild spring and/or warm autumn can mean a solid six or seven months of tick season. Take precautionary measures, but don't let ticks keep you inside your tent. Generally speaking, Lyme disease tends to be overdiagnosed and afflicts relatively few people.

Poison Ivy

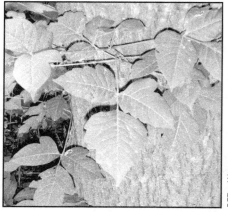

The old maxim for poison ivy holds true: "Leaves of three, let it be." Poison sumac, however, can contain anywhere from 7 to 13 leaves. Because I am extremely allergic to poison ivy, I always take the following precautions: I do not scratch anything under any circumstances; if poison ivy is sitting on the skin, scratching and then touching skin anywhere else is the surest way of spreading it. I carry alcohol-based moist towelettes, and at the end of the day, I rub my legs gently with the towelettes to stave off infection until I can get home and shower. (*Note:* It is very important that these moist towelettes contain alcohol. If they contain just soap, wiping with them will only move the poison ivy oil, urushiol, around, increasing the risk of infection.)

Mosquitoes

Many of the campgrounds in Southern Maryland and the Eastern Shore are simply inundated with mosquitoes in the humid summer months. Protect yourself against mosquito bites by applying an effective repellent. Most people reach for repellents that contain DEET, which is fairly toxic stuff. I prefer Burt's Bees natural insect repellent. I once took it with me on a trip into the Amazon jungle and found it very effective even there. Unlike DEET-based repellents, there is no maximum on the amount and frequency of use for Burt's.

:: RESOURCES

As you read this book, you'll see that the vast majority of the campgrounds are run by the Maryland Department of Natural Resources. I found time and time again that state-operated campgrounds were invariably clean, safe, and beautifully maintained. The Maryland DNR maintains an excellent website with links to all of the DNR-operated campgrounds featured in this book (33 of the 50). Visit **dnr2.maryland.gov** for all the latest information and links. *Note:* All DNR parks now include a per-night service charge in addition to the campground base rate. The service charges are as follows: online reservations, $4.56 per night; phone, $4.61 per night; on-site, $4.51 per night.

For information on private campgrounds in Maryland (including many not featured in this book), contact the Maryland Association of Campgrounds at 301-271-7012, or visit **mdcamping.com**.

:: TIPS FOR A HAPPY CAMPING TRIP

There is nothing worse than a bad camping trip, especially because it is so easy to have a great time. To assist with making your outing a happy one, here are some pointers:

- **Reserve your site ahead of time,** especially if it's a weekend or a holiday, or if the campground is wildly popular. Many prime campgrounds require significant lead time on reservations. Check before you go.

- **Pick your camping buddies wisely.** A family trip is pretty straightforward, but you may want to reconsider including grumpy Uncle Fred, who doesn't like bugs, sunshine, or marshmallows. After you know who's going, be sure everyone is on the same page regarding expectations of difficulty (amenities or the lack thereof, physical exertion, and so on), sleeping arrangements, and food requirements.

- **Don't duplicate equipment,** such as cooking pots and lanterns, among campers in your party. Carry what you need to have a good time, but don't turn the trip into a major moving experience.

- **Dress for the season.** Educate yourself on the temperature highs and lows of the specific area you plan to visit. It may be warm at night in the summer in your backyard, but it will be quite chilly up in the mountains.

- **Pitch your tent on a level surface,** preferably one covered with leaves, pine straw, or grass. Use a tarp or specially designed footprint to thwart ground moisture and to protect the tent floor. Do a little site maintenance, such as picking up the small rocks and sticks that can damage your tent floor and make sleep uncomfortable. If you have a separate tent rain fly but don't think you'll need it, keep it rolled up at the base of the tent in case it starts raining at midnight.

- **Take a sleeping pad.** If you are not comfortable sleeping on the ground, invest in a sleeping pad that is full-length and thicker than you think you might need. This will not only keep your hips from aching on hard ground, but will also help keep you warm. A wide range of thin, light, inflatable pads is available at camping stores, and these are a much better choice than home air mattresses, which conduct heat away from the body and tend to deflate during the night.

- **Don't skimp on food.** If you're not hiking into a primitive campsite, there is no real need to skimp on food due to weight. Plan tasty meals and bring everything you will need to prepare, cook, eat, and clean up.

- **If you tend to use the bathroom multiple times at night, plan ahead.** Leaving a warm sleeping bag and stumbling around in the dark to find the restroom, whether it be a pit toilet, a fully plumbed comfort station, or just the woods, is not fun. Keep a flashlight and any other accoutrements you may need by the tent door and know exactly where to head in the dark.

- **Watch out for standing dead trees and storm-damaged living trees.** These trees can pose a real hazard to tent campers, as they may have loose or broken limbs that could fall at any time. When choosing a campsite or even just a spot to rest during a hike, look up.

:: CAMPING ETIQUETTE

Camping experiences can vary wildly depending on a variety of factors, such as weather, preparedness, fellow campers, and time of year. Here are a few tips on how to create good vibes with fellow campers and wildlife you encounter.

- **Obtain all permits and authorizations as required.** Make sure you check in, pay your fee, and mark your site as directed. Don't make the mistake of grabbing a seemingly empty site that looks more appealing than your site. It could be reserved. If you're unhappy with the site you've selected, check with the campground host for other options.

- **Leave only footprints.** Be sensitive to the ground beneath you. Be sure to place all garbage in designated receptacles or pack it out if none is available. No one likes to see the trash someone else has left behind.

- **Never spook animals.** It's common for animals to wander through campsites, where they may be accustomed to the presence of humans (and our food). An unannounced approach, a sudden movement, or a loud noise will startle most animals. A surprised animal can be dangerous to you, to others, and to itself. Give animals plenty of space.

- **Plan ahead.** Know your equipment, your ability, and the area where you are camping and prepare accordingly. Be self-sufficient at all times; carry necessary supplies for changes in weather or other conditions. A well-executed trip is a satisfaction to you and to others.

- **Be courteous to other campers, hikers, bikers, and others you encounter.** If you run into the owner of a large RV, don't panic. Just wave, feign eye contact, and then walk away slowly.

- **Follow the campground's rules regarding the building of fires.** Never burn trash. Trash smoke smells horrible, and trash debris in a fire pit or grill is unsightly.

- **Everyone likes a fire, but bringing your own firewood from home is now frowned upon** by most campground operators. Bringing in wood from out of the area could introduce pests that are harmful to the forest. Use deadfall found near your campsite or purchase wood at the camp store.

:: VENTURING AWAY FROM THE CAMPGROUND

If you go for a hike, bike, or other excursion into the wilderness, here are some tips:

- **Always carry food and water,** whether you are planning to go overnight or not. Food will give you energy, help keep you warm, and sustain you in an emergency until help arrives. Bring potable water or treat water by boiling or filtering before drinking from a lake or stream.

- **Stay on designated trails.** Most hikers get lost when they leave the trail. Even on clearly marked trails, there is usually a point where you have to stop and consider which direction to head. If you become disoriented, don't panic. As soon as you think you may be off-track, stop, assess your current direction, and then retrace your steps back to the point where you went awry. If you have absolutely no idea how to continue, return to the trailhead the way you came in. Should you become completely lost and have no idea of how to return to the trailhead, remaining in place along the trail and waiting for help is most often the best option for adults and always the best option for children.

- **Be especially careful when crossing streams.** Whether you are fording the stream or crossing on a log, make every step count. If you have any doubt about maintaining your balance on a log, go ahead and ford the stream instead. When fording a stream, use a trekking pole or stout stick for balance and face upstream as you cross. If a stream seems too deep to ford, turn back. Whatever is on the other side is not worth risking your life.

- **Be careful at overlooks.** Although these areas may provide spectacular views, they are potentially hazardous. Stay back from the edge of outcrops and be absolutely sure of your footing: a misstep can mean a nasty and possibly fatal fall.

- **Know the symptoms of hypothermia.** Shivering and forgetfulness are the two most common indicators of this insidious killer. Hypothermia can occur at any elevation, even in the summer. Wearing cotton clothing puts you especially at risk, because cotton, when wet, wicks heat away from the body. To prevent hypothermia, dress in layers using synthetic clothing for insulation, use a cap and gloves to reduce heat loss, and protect yourself with waterproof, breathable outerwear. If symptoms arise, get the victim to a shelter with a fire, hot liquids, and dry clothes or a dry sleeping bag.

- **Take along your brain.** A cool, calculating mind is the single most important piece of equipment you'll ever need on the trail. Think before you act. Watch your step. Plan ahead. Avoiding accidents before they happen is the best recipe for a rewarding and relaxing hike.

Western Maryland

1

Big Run State Park

Big Run is just one of the many state parks and forests in Garrett County; what sets it apart from its neighbors is its proximity to the unspoiled Savage River Reservoir.

At **300 acres,** Big Run State Park is relatively modest in size, but it sits within the Savage River State Forest, which, at 53,000 acres, is the largest of Maryland's state forests and parks. Big Run is just one of the many state parks and forests in Garrett County; what sets it apart from its neighbors is its proximity to the unspoiled Savage River Reservoir, where anglers can fish for a seemingly endless supply of bass, catfish, crappie, perch, trout, and walleye. Fishing is permitted year-round with a nontidal fishing license.

Another feature that distinguishes Big Run from its larger park neighbor, New Germany, is that camping here is year-round. Because of the cold and the

:: Ratings

BEAUTY: ★ ★ ★ ★
PRIVACY: ★ ★ ★
QUIET: ★ ★ ★
SPACIOUSNESS: ★ ★ ★ ★
SECURITY: ★ ★ ★ ★ ★
CLEANLINESS: ★ ★ ★ ★ ★

threat of heavy snow, winter camping is largely a private experience. The numerous hiking trails in the state forest provide for some great cross-country skiing.

If you've brought a boat, you'll want to snag one of the sites in the 80s or sites 78, 79, or 90, which are closest to the boat launch for the reservoir. The closest two are 83 and 84. These are fairly big sites, but they are situated in an open grassy field without shade. In fact, all of sites 78–90 are in the open. If you wish for a wooded site, go with 60–75. If you are more interested in the surrounding forest and its hiking trails, go for the sites north of the boat launch, off Big Run Road (also sites 60–75). Sites 61 and 62 are closest to the lovely Monroe Run Trail. Be aware that sites 71 and 72 are closest to the Youth Group camping site, so the chance for noise is increased there.

Monroe Run Trail commences between sites 62 and 64, and these sites, along with 65 and 67, could be the most pleasurable spots to have. They sit in the forested sections of the park, away from the main camp roads. The trail follows

:: Key Information

ADDRESS: Big Run State Park
10368 Savage River Road
Swanton, MD 21561

CONTACT: 301-895-5453;
dnr2.maryland.gov

OPERATED BY: Maryland Department
of Natural Resources

OPEN: Year-round

SITES: 29

EACH SITE: Picnic table, fire grill,
lantern post

ASSIGNMENT: First come, first served

**REGISTRATION: reservations.dnr
.state.md.us** or 888-432-2267.
Self-registration station is located in the
lower camping area, along Savage
River Rd.

FACILITIES: Picnic pavilion, restroom,
water

PARKING: Maximum 2 vehicles/site

FEE: $10/night; $60/night group site
(25 people maximum)

RESTRICTIONS

- **Pets:** Allowed on a leash
- **Quiet Hours:** 11 p.m.–7 a.m.
- **Visitors:** Maximum 6 people/site
- **Fires:** In fire rings
- **Alcohol:** Permitted only inside
cabins and at shelters with valid
permit, as applicable
- **Stay Limit:** 2 weeks
- **Other:** Checkout 3 p.m.

Monroe Run into nearby New Germany State Park (see pages 71–73) and shouldn't be missed; it's a modest 6 miles, but it winds through pristine forests and over innumerable streams. It guarantees a workout, but it's lovely.

In all, you really can't go wrong in Big Run; it's fairly small, so there's really not a whole lot of action, company, or noise. And if you want an even more rustic camping experience, you can head straight north on Big Run Road or east on Savage River Road for loads of camping opportunities in the Savage River State Forest (see pages 85–92).

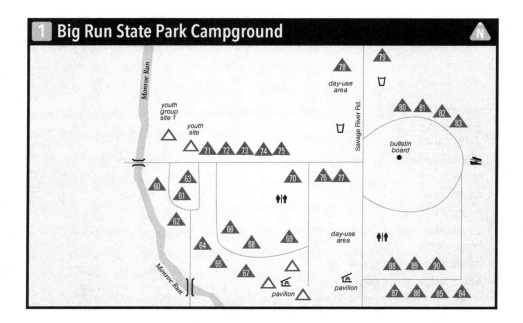

:: Getting There

Take Exit 22 off I-68 and follow Chestnut Ridge Road south to New Germany Road. Pass New Germany State Park headquarters and take a left onto Big Run Road. Go 5 miles, and the park is at the intersection of Big Run Road and Savage River Road.

GPS COORDINATES N39°32'42" W79°8'14"

2

Brunswick Family Campground

Brunswick Family Campground possesses some prime real estate astride a particularly beautiful stretch of the Potomac River.

Brunswick is a small city (population 5,000) in southwestern Frederick County, near the Washington County border. It's on the National Register of Historic Places because of its importance in the early to mid-1900s as a railroading town. The city also bumps up against the C&O Canal and the Potomac River. This wonderful location is what makes Brunswick Family Campground worth a visit. The campground itself used to be an airfield, so there's lots of space.

I must acknowledge, however, that I really debated whether or not I should include Brunswick Family Campground in the first edition of this book, and I debated again whether to include it in the second edition. Of the 50 campgrounds I've described here, I would rank it near the bottom. For one thing, it's primarily an RV campground. Additionally, in the first edition, I wrote the following: ". . . while the grounds are well maintained, the basketball court and, more important, the bathhouse (only one on site), are not." The good news: These facilities have been updated rather nicely, probably as a result of being under new management since 2012. But why did I ultimately decide to include it, yet again? Location, location, location.

Brunswick Family Campground possesses some prime real estate, astride a particularly beautiful stretch of the Potomac River. The same can be said of several other campsites in this book, most notably the C&O Canal drive-in and hiker-biker sites. However, the advantage that Brunswick Family Campground has over those is that you won't have to haul your gear to get there, and you're generally assured of getting a spot. Plus, the campground is less than a mile down a dirt road from the center of town and its

:: Ratings

BEAUTY: ★ ★
PRIVACY: ★
SPACIOUSNESS: ★ ★
QUIET: ★ ★
SECURITY: ★ ★ ★ ★ ★
CLEANLINESS: ★ ★ ★ ★

:: Key Information

ADDRESS: Brunswick Family Camp-ground, 100 S. Maple Avenue Brunswick, MD 21716

CONTACT: 301-695-5177; **potomacrivercampground.com**

OPERATED BY: Privately operated

OPEN: End of March–mid-November; weekends only April–Memorial Day

SITES: 100+

EACH SITE: Fire ring, picnic table

ASSIGNMENT: 301-834-9950 or check in at campground until 9 p.m. After 9 p.m., set up and pay in the morning.

REGISTRATION: Reserve by phone or just show up (see "Assignment" above).

FACILITIES: Ball fields, bathhouse, boat ramp, dumping station, play-ground, vending

PARKING: In designated areas

FEE: $9.52 plus 5% amusement fee; $4.76 plus 5% amusement fee/ages 12 and under; $2 off for handicapped, military, and seniors age 60 and older

RESTRICTIONS

▥ **Pets:** On a leash

▥ **Quiet Hours:** 10 p.m.–7 a.m.

▥ **Visitors:** Requested to stop by office and sign in

▥ **Fires:** In fire pits

▥ **Alcohol:** Permitted only inside cab-ins and at shelters with valid permit

▥ **Stay Limit:** 2-week limit/month but must wait at least 7 days between each 14-day stay

▥ **Other:** Check-in 3 p.m.; checkout 11 a.m. Campground is close to the CSX rail tracks and trains do come through.

most notable attraction, the Brunswick Railroad Museum, which also houses the C&O Canal National Historic Park Visitor Center for nearby Canal Lock 30. Furthermore, the campground enjoys proximity to state parks (Gathland and Gambrills); Civil War battlefields (Mono-cacy and the can't-miss Antietam, site of the largest battle of the war); and Harpers Ferry, West Virginia. As a result, it could provide for a nice family outing. There is often musical entertainment on week-ends (the campground has played host to the annual Shenandoah Riverside Festi-val in June, for example) when the camp-ground is full. Most of the campers are

locals, and Brunswick enjoys a reputation for friendliness.

My recommendation is to use the campground as a midweek destination for boating or fishing. I initially visited on a gorgeous Tuesday in June, and the place was virtually empty. There's a convenient boat ramp just beyond the entrance road.

Tent-only sites are spread through-out the campground, both left and right of the entrance. There is one tent site that is absolutely fantastic, and if you can get it, your experience should be quite spe-cial. All the way to the left when you enter, beyond sites 1–20 in RV Sections A and D, sit the Riverside tent sites in a little copse

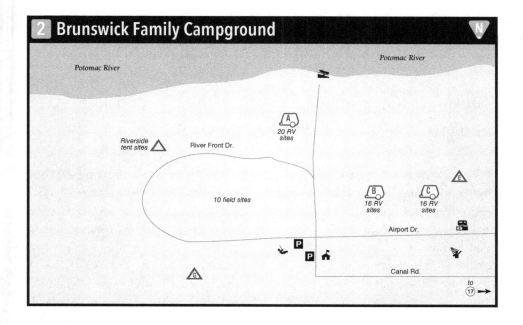

right in front of the river, with a small path heading off to the woods on the left. It's very private and spacious. It's one of the nicest spots you'll get anywhere, not just in this campground. There are other tent sites that aren't bad, though they are across the campground from the river, just to the left of the basketball court when you enter, toward the tree line.

The other tent-only sites sit to the right of the entrance on Airport Drive, just beyond RV Section C. The farther you head to the right, the farther you get from the RVs. However, moving farther to the right also brings you closer to the waste-treatment plant that looms just over the campground boundary. If you get too close, you will most likely smell it. Try to get a site closer to Section C so you won't see or smell the plant. Plus, this area is actually pretty nice and thickly wooded (though not very private).

:: Getting There

From Frederick, take I-70 to US 340 West to Exit 2, MD 17 South. Take A Street over the railroad tracks and then head left on the dirt road.

GPS COORDINATES   N39°18'25.8" W77°36'55.8"

3

Catoctin Mountain Park

Franklin D. Roosevelt was the first to use Catoctin as a presidential getaway, naming it Shangri-La.

Catoctin Mountain Park has a pedigreed history as a getaway spot— the presidential retreat at Camp David lies on the same property. The area was developed in the 1930s partly as a retreat for the families of federal employees. Although people are still fond of saying that D.C.'s population changes every election year and that no one actually lives there, those of us who grew up in and around D.C. know otherwise. We also know that summer—a time when it feels like the rest of the world is coming into the city—can be brutally hot and humid. Thus, a place like Catoctin, not too far away even in those days before mass transport and reliable, paved roads, is truly a retreat.

Franklin D. Roosevelt was the first to use Catoctin as a presidential getaway

:: Ratings

BEAUTY: ★ ★ ★ ★ ★
PRIVACY: ★ ★ ★ ★
SPACIOUSNESS: ★ ★ ★
QUIET: ★ ★ ★ ★
SECURITY: ★ ★ ★ ★ ★
CLEANLINESS: ★ ★ ★ ★ ★

in 1942. He named it Shangri-La. When Roosevelt died, some controversy arose over whether the land would remain in federal hands or revert to Maryland state parkland. A compromise was reached whereby the land north of MD 77 would remain under federal control, while the land south would go back to Maryland. (This southern area is now Cunningham Falls State Park; see pages 37–42.) The deal became official in 1954; soon after, President Eisenhower renamed the retreat after his grandson.

Obviously, a visitor to Catoctin Park shouldn't expect to be able to do any snooping around Camp David. In fact, chances are, you won't even know where it is in relation to where you're hiking or camping. (That said, I've been camping here when helicopters busily ferried dignitaries to and from the retreat.) The sections of the park that aren't off-limits contain more than 5,800 acres and more than 25 miles of hiking trails. Adding adjacent Cunningham Falls State Park, there's no shortage of recreational opportunities.

Catoctin's Owens Creek Campground sits near its namesake, the clean and clear Owens Creek. Several hiking trails also

:: Key Information

ADDRESS: Catoctin Mountain Park
6602 Foxville Road
Thurmont, MD 21788-1598

CONTACT: 301-663-9330;
nps.gov/cato

OPERATED BY: National Park Service

OPEN: May–November

SITES: 50

EACH SITE: Picnic table, grill, lantern post, tent pad

ASSIGNMENT: First come, first served

REGISTRATION: recreation.gov or 877-444-6777

FACILITIES: Bathhouse

PARKING: Only 1 vehicle at individual site; limited overflow parking

FEE: $25/night

RESTRICTIONS

▨ **Pets:** On a leash

▨ **Quiet Hours:** 10 p.m.–6 a.m.

▨ **Visitors:** Maximum 5 people or the immediate household/site

▨ **Fires:** In fire rings

▨ **Alcohol:** Permitted only inside cabins and at shelters with valid permit

▨ **Stay Limit:** No more than 7 consecutive days, or 14 days in a year

▨ **Other:** Maximum tent size 9x12 feet; checkout noon

come quite close, including the Catoctin Trail, which runs all the way through the park, into Cunningham Falls State Park, and farther south through the Frederick Municipal Forest. Nearer the park headquarters, it's easy to access trails that take in Chimney Rock, Wolf Rock, Thurmont Vista, and the Blue Ridge Summit Overlook, a fantastic loop through hardwood forests with grand, sweeping views.

I tend to have a bias toward the last site on any loop because of its minimal through traffic. For Catoctin, this is site 30, which sits virtually by itself at the end of the loop. If access to the bathhouse and water is most important to you, try to snag site 10 or 20. But the sites nearest Owens Creek are the most popular, and justly so—it's a lovely little tributary,

and the sites are very close to the creek. Essentially, the sites to the left of the entrance area—sites 1, 2, 4, 7, 14–16, 18, and 28–30—head toward the creek. Of these, sites 18, 28, and 29 are the best, with 30 a good bet as well because of its additional proximity to hiking trails.

Outside of the main campground loop, there are also two Adirondack shelters where you can camp; these are 3 miles downhill from the park. These primitive sites are lovely and provide nice space and privacy. These shelters are free, but permits are required (obtainable through the recreation.gov website). Tents must be set up inside the shelters. The shelters can accommodate five people and provide access to a pit toilet. They both sit within 3 miles of parking areas.

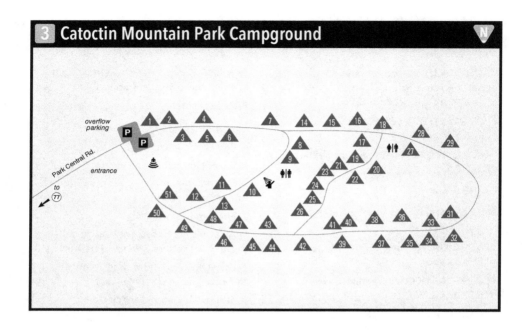

:: Getting There

From Frederick, take US 15 17 miles north to Thurmont. Take MD 77 West. Go 3 miles and turn right onto Park Central Road.

GPS COORDINATES N39°39'11.2" W77°27'49.6"

4

C&O Canal: Drive-In Sites

All campsites along the canal have two things in common: the Potomac in front and the towpath behind.

The **C&O Canal** follows the Potomac River for 185 miles from Washington, D.C., to Cumberland, Maryland. It functioned for almost 100 years beginning in 1828, and a multitude of original structures still stand, attesting to its durability and workmanship. It came close to becoming a highway, but through the tireless efforts of Supreme Court Justice William O. Douglas in the mid-1950s, it was turned instead into a linear park in 1971. Today, we are the beneficiaries. I recommend checking out **canaltrust .org/trust,** the website of the C&O Canal Trust, the nonprofit partner of the Historic Trust, which offers loads of wonderful info on sites along the canal.

The C&O Canal enjoys a reputation as the best-preserved 19th-century canal in America, and restoration projects continue to this day. Potomac floods periodically wash away major portions of the canal, so restoration will probably go on perpetually. Like the monuments and museums in D.C., the canal's mission is a public one. To that end, a whole series of hiker-biker campsites are set up and maintained and are free of charge (see the next three profiles in this book).

There are also five drive-in campsites along the C&O Canal, none of which have electrical hookups. In choosing where to go and what to see along the canal, you have to familiarize yourself with the numbering system. Everything along the canal is assigned a number according to its distance from Mile 0, at the canal's starting point at the Georgetown Visitor Center in Washington, D.C.

The five drive-in sites are spread along the canal but are more along the northwestern sections toward Cumberland (as opposed to southeast toward Washington). They are Antietam Creek (Mile 70), McCoys Ferry (Mile 110), Fifteen Mile Creek (Mile 141), Paw Paw (Mile 156), and Spring Gap (Mile 173).

All campsites along the canal have two things in common: the Potomac

:: Ratings

BEAUTY: ★ ★ ★ ★
PRIVACY: ★ ★
QUIET: ★ ★ ★ ★
SPACIOUSNESS: ★ ★ ★ ★
SECURITY: ★ ★ ★ ★
CLEANLINESS: ★ ★ ★ ★

:: Key Information

ADDRESS: C&O Canal NHP Headquarters, 1850 Dual Highway, Suite 100 Hagerstown, MD 21740-6620

CONTACT: 301-739-4200; **nps.gov/choh**

OPERATED BY: National Park Service

OPEN: Year-round

SITES: 5 locations, 71 sites total

EACH SITE: Picnic table, fire pit

ASSIGNMENT: First come, first served

REGISTRATION: Self-registration at each site; pay before occupying site

FACILITIES: Chemical toilets, grills, water (except McCoys Ferry)

PARKING: Maximum 2 vehicles/site; park only at designated sites, never on grass. You must have a parking tag if you leave a car overnight at a canal parking lot; to access a registration form, visit: **nps.gov/choh**

FEE: $10/night

RESTRICTIONS

- **Pets:** On a leash or under control
- **Quiet Hours:** 10 p.m.–6 a.m.
- **Visitors:** Maximum 8 people or 2 tents/site
- **Fires:** In grills or fire rings only
- **Alcohol:** Not allowed
- **Stay Limit:** Total of 30 days for the calendar year, only 14 of which can be consecutive or between May 1 and October 1

in front and the towpath behind. This means endless opportunities for boating, fishing, swimming, and hiking. Each drive-in campground is somewhat different in character, however, in that the surrounding topography changes and nearby historical sites and towns (or lack thereof) change the experience of camping in each site. As a general rule, expect large, cleared areas with individual campsites scattered around the available space. While the sites are usually big, they're never terribly far from one another. Antietam Creek's main draw is its proximity to Antietam National Battlefield, which is a short drive (or canoe ride) away. Antietam is hallowed ground, site of the bloodiest battle in the Civil War. Excellent maintenance and educational opportunities distinguish the park. But it's also an exceedingly beautiful place, and a canoe or kayak trip upstream through the battlefield site is a special experience. Take MD 34 West to Sharpsburg and go south on S. Mechanic Street, which soon turns into Harpers Ferry Road. Go 3 miles to the campground. There are 20 campsites at Antietam Creek, and water is available between mid-April and mid-November.

McCoys Ferry tends to be more popular, as it has RV parking. As mentioned previously, there are no electric sites at any of the C&O Canal campgrounds, but RVs in the area can use this parking lot. McCoys Ferry is also popular because it has a boat ramp for quick launch into the Potomac.

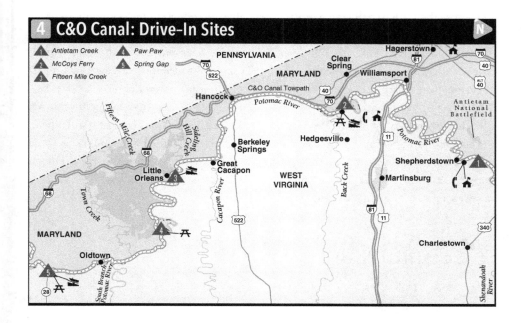

4 C&O Canal: Drive-In Sites

1 Antietam Creek
2 McCoys Ferry
3 Fifteen Mile Creek
4 Paw Paw
5 Spring Gap

PENNSYLVANIA

MARYLAND

WEST VIRGINIA

MARYLAND

The launch parking lot is where you have to leave your car. Be aware that there is no potable water at this site. McCoys Ferry has 14 sites and is nicely situated just south of Fort Frederick State Park (see pages 47–49) and Big Pool. To reach McCoys Ferry, take I-70 to Exit 12 and follow MD 56 past Big Pool and Fort Frederick. Take a right onto McCoys Ferry Road.

Fifteen Mile Creek, with 10 sites, also has parking and a boat launch. There is water available between mid-April and mid-November. If you need other supplies, the town of Little Orleans is nearby. The campsite sits on the southern edge of Green Ridge State Forest (see pages 59–64), so if the level terrain of the canal gets tiresome, you can head for the forested hills. A bit farther out, back on I-68, is the Sideling Hill Visitor Center.

The four-story center sits perched atop one of the most dramatic rock exposures in the eastern U.S. When the highway was blasted through the mountain, it exposed almost 850 feet of vertical rock layers formed some 350 million years ago. To reach Fifteen Mile Creek, take I-68 to Exit 68 and follow Orleans Road south 11 miles to a left on High Germany Road.

Paw Paw may be the canal's most popular site. The chief attraction here is the Paw Paw Tunnel, a 3,100-foot-long tunnel constructed between 1836 and 1850. Paw Paw allows easy access to Green Ridge State Forest, entering from the west side. Paw Paw campground, with eight sites, is loaded with amenities. Aside from parking and a boat launch, there are picnic areas, phones, and a camp store and restaurants nearby, just across the bridge in the town of Paw Paw, West Virginia. To reach the Paw Paw camping area, pick up Oldtown Orleans Road SE in Little Orleans (see directions to Fifteen Mile Creek above) to MD 51, and head south.

The amenities listed for Paw Paw are also found at Spring Gap (sans the restaurants), the westernmost drive-in campground, with 19 sites. This is a more remote section of the canal, sitting in the shadow of Warrior Mountain (what a great name!) and within 10 miles of the canal's terminus at Cumberland. Spring Gap is 18 miles west of Paw Paw on MD 51. There is no water here.

Note: Group sites can hold up to 35, require reservations (call the park office), and are located at Marsden Tract (Mile 11), adjacent to the drive-in site at Fifteen Mile Creek (Mile 141).

:: Getting There

Varies; see text.

GPS COORDINATES
Antietam Creek: N39°25'07.1" W77°44'39.0"
McCoys Ferry: N39°36'28.4" W77°58'08.5"
Fifteen Mile Creek: N39°37'25.6" W78°23'10.3"
Paw Paw: N39°32'39.1" W78°27'41.4"
Spring Gap: N39°33'52.5" W78°43'05.3"

5

C&O Canal: Hiker-Biker Campsites from Swain's Lock (Mile 16.6) to Killiansburg Cave (Mile 75.2)

In virtually every case, the campsites sit along the Potomac and the C&O in wooded copses.

There are 32 tent-only hiker-biker campsites along the canal, located roughly every 5 miles. Hiker-biker sites are limited to one night per site. This can be an annoyance for many, as it requires breaking down and cleaning up daily. However, it creates a great situation for people who want to hike, bike, or boat their way along a segment of the river and canal. My buddy Jack and I once kayaked from Paw Paw, West Virginia, down to Hancock, Maryland, and the campsites along the way were perfectly suited for our needs.

The hiker-biker sites are often physically indistinguishable from one another, so determining which one you want comes down to location: In virtually every case, they sit along the Potomac and the C&O

:: Ratings

BEAUTY: ★ ★ ★ ★
PRIVACY: ★ ★ ★ ★
QUIET: ★ ★ ★ ★
SPACIOUSNESS: ★ ★ ★ ★
SECURITY: ★ ★ ★ ★
CLEANLINESS: ★ ★ ★ ★

in wooded copses. What I mean here about location is distance from wherever you're traveling and distance from where you'll have to leave your car. In some cases, there's a decent hike required to get to the site from the nearest parking area. This has an advantage in that the farther you go, the greater the chances of solitude. Of course, if you're hauling a lot of gear, it might be nice to have a quick walk from the car.

The C&O Canal is popular in many places; expect hikers and bikers passing by your site at all hours of the day. Some people worry that their belongings are easily accessed by others while they're, say, out on the river. This is a legitimate concern. However, I've never spoken to one camper who has had an experience of thievery while camping along the C&O Canal.

Officially, swimming is prohibited in the canal, as well as in the Potomac where it borders D.C. and Montgomery County. This means everything south of the Indian Flats hiker-biker site—for this entry, that covers Swains Lock, Horsepen Branch, Chisel Branch, Turtle Run, and Marble Quarry—so if swimming in the river is

:: Key Information

ADDRESS: C&O Canal NHP Headquarters, 1850 Dual Highway, Suite 100 Hagerstown, MD 21740

CONTACT: 301-739-4200; nps.gov/choh

OPERATED BY: National Park Service

OPEN: Year-round

SITES: 10

EACH SITE: Grill, chemical toilet, picnic table, pump well water (but plan for the possibility of a pump not working)

ASSIGNMENT: First come, first served

REGISTRATION: None

FACILITIES: Varies by site; see text

PARKING: Vehicles must be left at the nearest parking area; see text for individual sites

FEE: Free

RESTRICTIONS

▧ **Pets:** None

▧ **Quiet Hours:** None

▧ **Visitors:** Maximum 8 people/site

▧ **Fires:** In fire rings or portable grills only

▧ **Alcohol:** Not allowed

▧ **Stay Limit:** 1 night/site/trip

▧ **Other:** Only dead wood can be collected for fires.

your primary goal in camping along the canal, head farther northwest. These sites include Indian Flats, Calico Rocks, Bald Eagle Island, Huckleberry Hill, and Killiansburg Cave in this entry and all the other sites in the following two entries in this book. The National Park Service doesn't recommend swimming anywhere in the river, as currents can be deceptively strong. However, swimming near the shore and taking due caution is usually safe.

Generally speaking, each hiker-biker site is just one cleared area where folks can pitch a tent. The amount of cleared space corresponds to the popularity of the area. The first hiker-biker site is at Mile 16.6, at Swains Lock. This is a very popular area, with phones, food, and bike and boat rentals nearby. There's a lot of camping space here, as this could be the most heavily trafficked area on the entire

canal. A major reason for that is Great Falls, 2.5 miles downstream. Great Falls is beautiful and the best place to see the Potomac at its most awesome as it roils through serrated rocks. It's also popular with hikers taking on the Billy Goat Trail and exploring Mather Gorge. To get to Swains Lock, take I-495 to River Road West (Exit 39) and then turn left about a quarter mile past Piney Meetinghouse Road onto Swains Lock Road.

Horsepen Branch hiker-biker (Mile 26.1) sits on the edge of the McKee-Beshers Wildlife Management Area (2,000 acres) and is just north of Seneca Creek State Park (6,300 acres), so hikers have it good. From I-270, take MD 109 south, and then take West Willard Road until it ends at Sycamore Landing. You can park at the boat launch there and then walk south (downstream) for 1 mile.

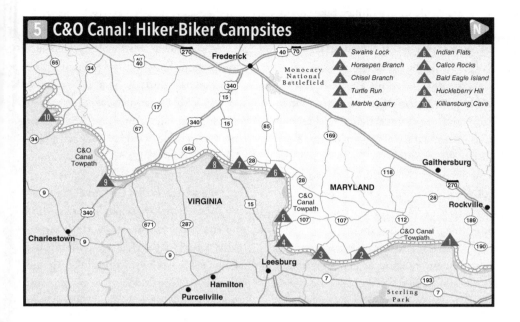

At Chisel Branch (Mile 30.5), things begin to feel a bit more remote; the day crowds dry up and there's a sense of wildness. Follow the directions above to Horsepen Branch; but, on West Willard Road, take a right toward Edwards Ferry and park there. The hiker-biker campsite is 0.3 mile upstream. The lockhouse (1791–1836) just upstream at Edwards Ferry is still in great condition.

Turtle Run (Mile 34.4): This area is studded with culverts (no less than seven of them within a 2-mile span). Things go, temporarily, back to feeling a bit like they did closer to D.C. Because White's Ferry is still operating, this area attracts a lot of visitors. Take MD 109 to a right onto MD 107 North. Turtle Run is 1 mile south of MD 107. MD 107 leads to a toll ferry across the river to Leesburg, Virginia. You can park at the ferry and then walk

downstream 1.1 miles to Turtle Run. Marble Quarry (Mile 38.2) is similar to Turtle Run, only upstream instead of down. To get there, park at White's Ferry.

Indian Flats hiker-biker (Mile 42.5) is the first campsite where you are legally allowed to swim in the Potomac. Indian Flats sits roughly equidistant from two boat launches at Monocacy downstream and Nolands Ferry upstream. Take MD 109 south to MD 28 and head northwest toward Monocacy. Park at the Monocacy Aqueduct. Indian Flats is 0.3 mile upstream. Monocacy Aqueduct is the largest of the canal's aqueducts and is considered an engineering marvel and must-see.

Calico Rocks hiker-biker (Mile 47.6) is next. A word of warning about this site: An operable railroad is nearby, and it can get noisy, even during the night. From Frederick, take US 340 to US 15 to Point of Rocks. Calico Rocks hiker-biker is 0.5 mile downstream. The same issue with rail noise plagues the next hiker-biker site: Bald Eagle Island (Mile 50.3). Follow the same directions for Calico Rocks, but take MD 464 west to a left on Lander Road and park there. Bald Eagle Island hiker-biker is 0.6 mile downstream. Both Calico Rocks and Bald Eagle Island are near Frederick and Brunswick, so it's a quick and easy trip to civilization.

Between Bald Eagle Island and the next hiker-biker site, there's a big gap; this is filled by the city of Brunswick, the Appalachian Trail as it heads down South Mountain (in fact, the AT and the canal towpath are one and the same between Lock 31 and 32), and the river crossing for Harpers Ferry, where the Potomac and Shenandoah Rivers meet. At mile 62.9, you'll find Huckleberry Hill hiker-biker. This, like Seneca to the south, is a popular spot, mostly because of its proximity to Harpers Ferry. A word of warning: If you've come for boating, the waters just downstream, between Locks 32 and 34, are considered hazardous. Take MD 34 from Boonsboro to a left on Harpers Ferry Road crossing through Antietam, and follow the river south to Dargan. Park at Dargan Bend, and then walk 2 miles downstream.

Last is Killiansburg Cave (Mile 75.2), so called because of the small caves in the rock where locals sought shelter during the battle of Antietam. (In between is the Antietam Creek Drive-in Campsite, see pages 21–24.) Proximity to Antietam National Battlefield and a ranger station just downstream make Killiansburg a nice camping spot. Take MD 34 from Boonsboro, cross MD 65 at Sharpsburg, and take the first right toward the boat launch at Snyders Landing. Killiansburg Cave is approximately 1 mile downstream.

:: Getting There

Varies; see text.

GPS COORDINATES
Swains Lock: N39°01'52.8" W77°14'37.8"
Horsepen Branch: N39°04'12.0" W77°23'59.5"
Chisel Branch: N39°05'25.8" W77°27'47.4"
Turtle Run: N39°08'22.3" W77°30'56.0"
Marble Quarry: N39°10'46.6" W77°29'32.8"
Indian Flats: N39°13'50.3" W77°27'28.1"
Calico Rocks: N39°15'51.4" W77°31'19.6"
Bald Eagle Island: N39°17'56.3" W77°33'25.4"
Huckleberry Hill: N39°20'10.0" W77°44'45.8"
Killiansburg Cave: N39°27'26.5" W77°47'45.4"

6

C&O Canal: Hiker-Biker Campsites from Horseshoe Bend (Mile 79) to Cacapon Junction (Mile 133)

North Mountain is nicely wild, with little evidence of humanity, either modern or historical.

For general information on hiker-biker sites, read the introductory material in the previous profile. What follows is a continuation of those sites, moving northwesterly along the C&O Canal toward Cumberland.

After Antietam and Killiansburg Cave comes the Horseshoe Bend hiker-biker site (Mile 79.2). This area is closest to the city of Hagerstown, where you can get whatever supplies you need. From Hagerstown, take MD 65 south from I-70 about 8 miles to a right at Taylors Landing Road to the boat launch. Horseshoe Bend is 1.7 miles downstream.

:: Ratings

BEAUTY: ★ ★ ★ ★
PRIVACY: ★ ★ ★ ★
QUIET: ★ ★ ★ ★
SPACIOUSNESS: ★ ★ ★ ★
SECURITY: ★ ★ ★ ★
CLEANLINESS: ★ ★ ★ ★

Big Woods (Mile 82.7) shares the same parking as Horseshoe Bend but sits 1.6 miles downstream. The canal's midpoint is here, just before the next hiker-biker site, Opequon Junction, and Lock 43. The Big Woods hiker-biker campsite enjoys a reputation for privacy, as it sits down a little trail from the canal towpath, while most others sit just off the towpath. The area between Big Woods and the next upstream launch at Big Slackwater, at roughly Mile 87, is susceptible to erosion and damage from flooding, sometimes rendering portions of the towpath impassable, so be aware of that possibility. Opequon Junction (Mile 90.9) has parking 2 miles downstream at McMahons Mill. To get there from I-70, take Exit 28 and head southwest on MD 632 (Downsville Pike) 5.5 miles. Take a right onto Dellinger Road, and then the first left onto Avis Mill Road.

For the next hiker-biker site, Cumberland Valley (Mile 95.2), park 4.1 miles downstream at Williamsport, which has a visitor center, boat and bike rental,

:: Key Information

ADDRESS: C&O Canal NHP Headquarters, 1850 Dual Highway, Suite 100 Hagerstown, MD 21740-6620

CONTACT: 301-739-4200; nps.gov/choh

OPERATED BY: National Park Service

OPEN: Year-round

SITES: 11

EACH SITE: Grill, chemical toilet, picnic table, pump well water (but plan for the possibility of a pump not working)

ASSIGNMENT: First come, first served

REGISTRATION: None

FACILITIES: Varies by site; see text

PARKING: Vehicles must be left at the nearest parking area; see text for individual sites

FEE: Free

RESTRICTIONS

▓ **Pets:** None

▓ **Quiet Hours:** None

▓ **Visitors:** Maximum 8 people/site

▓ **Fires:** In fire rings or portable grills only

▓ **Alcohol:** Not allowed

▓ **Stay Limit:** 1 night/site/trip

▓ **Other:** Only dead wood can be collected for fires.

phone, picnic area, food (I recommend the Desert Rose Café), and a boat launch. Take I-70 to I-81 South and immediately exit onto US 11; travel south 3 miles to the river. Williamsport itself is worth a look around. Most Marylanders like to boast that Annapolis was once the national capital and is still America's oldest continuous state capital. But few Marylanders are aware that George Washington once considered tiny Williamsport for the national capital (it was rejected because it lacked a deep-water port). Loads of historical canal structures still stand in and around Williamsport. Jordan Junction hiker-biker site (Mile 101.2) also uses the parking area at Williamsport, 1.4 miles downstream. A word of warning if you're boating in this area: Dams above and at Williamsport mean you have to portage on the West Virginia side.

North Mountain hiker-biker site is next, at Mile 110. Parking is 0.4 mile upstream at McCoys Ferry, which is a drive-in campsite (see pages 22–23). The section between this campsite and the previous is nicely wild, with little evidence of humanity, either modern or historical. But just a couple of miles beyond North Mountain hiker-biker site is Fort Frederick, a 250-year-old treasure that is worth a half-day's poking around. (For information on camping at Fort Frederick, see pages 47–49). Then, things start to get rural again.

Next up is Licking Creek hiker-biker site (Mile 116). I wouldn't necessarily recommend it, as it sits very near I-70 and you can hear the traffic at night. In fact, the parking area for this campsite is adjacent to the I-70 exit ramp at Indian Springs (Exit 9), 0.7 mile upstream.

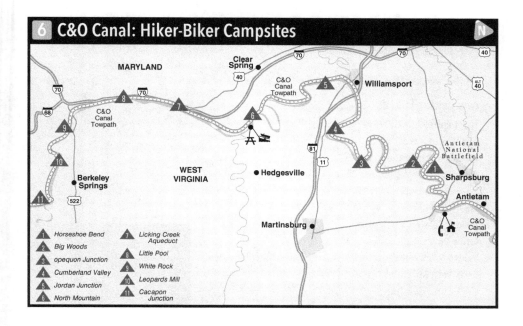

6 C&O Canal: Hiker-Biker Campsites

1. Horseshoe Bend
2. Big Woods
3. opequon Junction
4. Cumberland Valley
5. Jordan Junction
6. North Mountain
7. Licking Creek Aqueduct
8. Little Pool
9. White Rock
10. Leopards Mill
11. Cacapon Junction

The next four hiker-biker sites all share the same parking area at Little Tonoloway, which has a boat launch, restaurants, groceries, phone, and the visitor center in the town of Hancock. Unfortunately, the first of those four campsites, Little Pool (Mile 120.6), also sits right next to I-70. But if you can stand the noise, the site is 3.9 miles downstream of Little Tonoloway. To reach Little Tonoloway, take US 522 toward Hancock from I-70 (Exit 3) to W. Main Street in Hancock. Take the first right onto S. Pennsylvania Avenue.

White Rock hiker-biker site (Mile 126.4) is next. Just a mile upstream is what remains of the Round Top Cement Mill. While the redbrick mill remains only as an intact smokestack and some crumbling walls, the nearby kilns, eight

of them total, still look great and are largely intact. By all means, check them out, but be aware of the three bat species (big brown, little brown, and Eastern pipistrelle) that hibernate there.

Leopards Mill hiker-biker site (Mile 129.9) is 5.4 miles upstream of Little Tonoloway, one of the longer hikes to reach a campsite in the C&O Canal system. But an even longer hike is the one to Cacapon Junction (Mile 133.6), which is a solid 6.8 miles upstream from Little Tonoloway—no terrible haul if you're on a bike, but a bit of a slog if you've got all your equipment on your back. Cacapon Junction is the area where the Cacapon River, a simply beautiful Potomac tributary, meets the Potomac on the West Virginia side.

:: Getting There

Varies; see text.

GPS COORDINATES
Horseshoe Bend: N39°28'16.5" W77°47'33.1"
Big Woods: N39°29'35.6" W77°47'28.3"
Opequon Junction: N39°31'08.4" W77°51'46.9"
Cumberland Valley: N39°33'41.4" W77°52'43.0"
Jordan Junction: N39°36'37.9" W77°51'42.2"
North Mountain: N39°36'17.9" W77°58'22.9"
Licking Creek Aqueduct: N39°40'14.7" W78°04'36.3"
Little Pool: N39°41'04.1" W78°06'38.2"
White Rock: N39°41'06.2" W78°11'49.4"
Leopards Mill: N39°39'42.5" W78°13'31.6"
Cacapon Junction: N39°37'18.9" W78°16'55.1"

7

C&O Canal: Hiker-Biker Campsites from Indigo Neck (Mile 139) to Evitts Creek (Mile 180)

The first five hiker-biker campsites in this section all sit within or adjacent to the Green Ridge State Forest.

For general information on hiker-biker sites, read "C&O Canal: Hiker-Biker Campsites from Swain's Lock (Mile 16.6) to Killiansburg Cave (Mile 75.2)" on pages 25–28. What follows is a continuation of those sites from Cacapon Junction (Mile 133), moving northwesterly along the C&O Canal toward Cumberland.

The first five hiker-biker campsites in this section all sit within or adjacent to the Green Ridge State Forest, which offers fantastic camping opportunities. (For a description of Green Ridge camping, see pages 59–64.) The first site, Indigo Neck (Mile 139.2), uses the parking area 1.6 miles upstream at Fifteen Mile Creek, which is a drive-in site (see pages 21–24). Sideling Hill Creek, a lovely little Potomac tributary that begins in Pennsylvania, is just south of the Indigo Neck hiker-biker site. To get to the parking area at Fifteen Mile Creek, take I-68 and exit at Little Orleans Road (Exit 68). Continue 5.5 miles south to a left onto High Germany Road.

Devil's Alley (Mile 144.5), the next hiker-biker site, also uses the parking area at Fifteen Mile Creek, this time 3.7 miles downstream.

Stickpile Hill (Mile 149.4) and Sorrel Ridge (Mile 154.1) hiker-biker sites are next; as mentioned above, they are all adjacent to the Green Ridge State Forest, which offers a tremendous amount of recreational activity.

After Sorrel Ridge, the towpath breaks up a bit just after Lock 62 as the river squiggles in a series of little bends. To continue hiking upstream toward Paw Paw Tunnel and Paw Paw drive-in campsite (see pages 21–24), you can take the Tunnel Hill Trail.

:: Ratings

BEAUTY: ★ ★ ★ ★
PRIVACY: ★ ★ ★ ★
QUIET: ★ ★ ★ ★
SPACIOUSNESS: ★ ★ ★ ★
SECURITY: ★ ★ ★ ★
CLEANLINESS: ★ ★ ★ ★

:: Key Information

ADDRESS: C&O Canal NHP Headquarters, 1850 Dual Highway, Suite 100 Hagerstown, MD 21740-6620

CONTACT: 301-739-4200; **nps.gov/choh**

OPERATED BY: National Park Service

OPEN: Year-round

SITES: 10

EACH SITE: Grill, chemical toilet, picnic table, pump well water (but plan for the possibility of a pump not working)

ASSIGNMENT: First come, first served

REGISTRATION: None

FACILITIES: Varies by site; see text

PARKING: Vehicles must be left at the nearest parking area; see text for individual sites.

FEE: Free

RESTRICTIONS

▓ **Pets:** None

▓ **Quiet Hours:** None

▓ **Visitors:** Maximum 8 people/site

▓ **Fires:** In fire rings or portable grills only

▓ **Alcohol:** Not allowed

▓ **Stay Limit:** 1 night/site/trip

▓ **Other:** Only dead wood can be collected for fires.

Use the Paw Paw campsite parking for both Stickpile Hill and Sorrel Ridge. For Stickpile, Paw Paw is 6.6 miles upstream, and for Sorrel, it's 1.9 miles upstream. To reach Paw Paw, take I-68 to Exit 62 into the Green Ridge Forest, on Green Ridge Road W. Head south on MD 51 just before Town Creek Aqueduct.

Purslane Run (Mile 157.4) is next, also using the Paw Paw parking area, this time 1.6 miles downstream. Aside from Green Ridge State Forest, the big attraction here is the Paw Paw Tunnel, by far the most impressive engineering marvel along the canal. Paw Paw Tunnel stretches 3,100 feet and was constructed between 1836 and 1850. The drive-in campsite at Paw Paw gives access to picnic areas, phones, a camp store, and nearby restaurants.

Town Creek Aqueduct (Mile 162.1) is the next hiker-biker campsite, sitting on the westernmost edge of the state forest. Town Creek runs just north of the state forest and empties into the Potomac just north of the campsite. To reach the Town Creek hiker-biker site, take I-68 to Exit 62 into the Green Ridge Forest on Green Ridge Road W. Because the road ends just before the campsite, the camping area can potentially feel a bit crowded. That said, this is not a major traffic thoroughfare by any stretch; in fact, because many of the forest roads are unpaved, the farther you get from I-68, the fewer people you see.

Where the two branches of the Potomac meet is where you'll find the next hiker-biker site, the aptly named Potomac Forks, at Mile 164.8. I find this

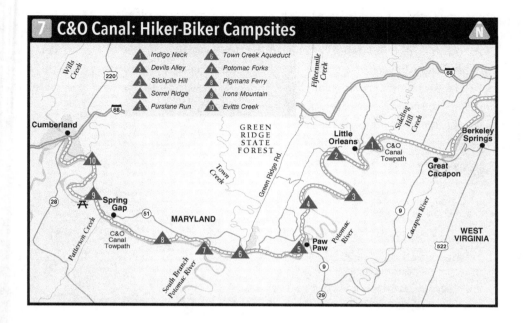

7 C&O Canal: Hiker-Biker Campsites

1. Indigo Neck
2. Devils Alley
3. Stickpile Hill
4. Sorrel Ridge
5. Purslane Run
6. Town Creek Aqueduct
7. Potomac Forks
8. Pigmans Ferry
9. Irons Mountain
10. Evitts Creek

to be an especially scenic spot, and it's one of my favorite campsites. Just to the north looms Warrior Mountain. At 2,185 feet, it's Maryland's seventh highest. Parking for Potomac Forks is 1.9 miles upstream, at Oldtown. To reach it, follow the directions above for Town Creek Aqueduct, but head north on MD 51. Once you hit Main Street, look for leftward turns toward the canal.

Pigmans Ferry hiker-biker site (Mile 169.1) also uses the parking areas in Oldtown, this time 1.4 miles downstream. The Spring Gap drive-in site is at Mile 173.3, where you can take advantage of many amenities; for a full description, see page 24.

Next up is Irons Mountain hiker-biker site (Mile 175.3). For Irons Mountain, use the parking area 2 miles

upstream. To reach it, take I-68 to Exit 43C in Cumberland to MD 51. Travel south 7 miles, turn right onto Pittsburgh Plate Glass Road, and then take the first left. Irons Mountain sits near a noisy railroad trestle, so be warned. Perhaps you'd be better off in the next hiker-biker site, Evitts Creek (Mile 180.1), the final campsite along the C&O Canal. Parking for Evitts Creek is 4.4 miles upstream at the Western Maryland Terminus, the end point for the canal towpath, in the town of Cumberland. There's a visitor center here, as well as bike rentals and groceries.

Cumberland itself is worth a day of poking around. I especially like the idea of parking here, spending some hours checking things out, and then walking or biking the 4.4 miles to the Evitts Creek campsite. Of course, I wouldn't be the only one with this idea, and it's not unreasonable to expect that the campsite, so close to a large town and the end of a line, may be occupied. *Note:* The sewage disposal plant at Mile 181.2 is rather unpleasant, but the smell dissipates quickly after leaving the plant behind. In truth, I would recommend heading a little farther east, as too many of Cumberland's nearby municipal necessities make this a not-too-wild and potentially unpleasant camping experience.

:: Getting There

Varies; see text.

GPS COORDINATES
Indigo Neck: N39°37'38.5" W78°21'38.3"
Devils Alley: N39°36'25.4" W78°25'47.0"
Stickpile Hill: N39°35'01.7" W78°23'52.9"
Sorrel Ridge: N39°34'16.8" W78°27'12.7"
Purslane Run: N39°31'12.8" W78°28'00.2"
Town Creek Aqueduct: N39°31'29.4" W78°32'51.4"
Potomac Forks: N39°31'50.0" W78°35'20.2"
Pigmans Ferry: N39°32'18.4" W78°38'25.5"
Irons Mountain: N39°35'13.8" W78°43'59.0"
Evitts Creek: N39°37'28.0" W78°44'20.3"

8

Cunningham Falls State Park:
Houck Area

The park's namesake is a 78-foot waterfall, which qualifies as Maryland's largest cascading waterfall.

Cunningham Falls State Park is situated in the Catoctin Mountains. The park's namesake is a 78-foot waterfall, which qualifies as Maryland's largest cascading waterfall. Franklin Roosevelt first used the area north of Cunningham Falls State Park as a presidential retreat in 1942, trying to escape the oppressive heat of D.C. summers. He named it Shangri-La. When Roosevelt died, there was some controversy over whether the land would remain in federal hands or revert to Maryland state parkland. A compromise was reached: North of MD 77 would remain under federal control, while land south, today's Cunningham Falls State Park, would go back to Maryland. Today, Cunningham Falls State Park has two separate camping sections: William Houck and Manor.

William Houck is by far the larger of the two campgrounds in the park. This is because it sits next to the park's main attractions: Hunting Creek Lake (with its boating and fishing) and Cunningham Falls. Hunting Creek Lake is a put-and-take trout area, with bass, bluegills, catfish, crappie, and sunfish. Big Hunting Creek, the lake's feeder, provides more fishing opportunities.

Cunningham Falls is an easy half-mile hike from the Houck camping area along the Falls Trail. The park itself has lots of hiking trails, including a mostly isolated one (part of the Catoctin Trail) heading to the Manor camping area. Additionally, the park's fluid border with Catoctin Mountain Park (see pages 18–20) ensures even more hiking opportunities nearby.

My favorite trail within the park is Cat Rock/Bob's Hill, which runs 7.5 miles across the mountain and takes in scenic rock outcrops. It's also easy to link this to Catoctin Mountain Park's trails to more

:: Ratings

BEAUTY: ★ ★ ★ ★ ★
PRIVACY: ★ ★ ★
SPACIOUSNESS: ★ ★ ★ ★
QUIET: ★ ★ ★
SECURITY: ★ ★ ★ ★ ★
CLEANLINESS: ★ ★ ★ ★ ★

:: Key Information

ADDRESS: Cunningham Falls State Park
14039 Catoctin Hollow Road
Thurmont, MD 21788

CONTACT: 301-271-7574;
dnr2.maryland.gov

OPERATED BY: Maryland Department
of Natural Resources

OPEN: Early April–late October

SITES: 138 (11 camper cabins)

EACH SITE: Picnic table, fire ring,
lantern post, tent pad

ASSIGNMENT: Reservations
recommended

REGISTRATION: 888-432-CAMP
(2267), **reservations.dnr.state.md.us,**
or at campground registration off
Catoctin Hollow Road. First come, first
served in April.

FACILITIES: Bathhouse, camp store,
boat launch, concessions, dump station,
playground, water

PARKING: In designated camp spots

FEE: $21.49 plus service charge/night,
$27.49 plus service charge/night elec-
tric; additional day-use service charge
during high season $3–$5

RESTRICTIONS

▓ **Pets:** Allowed in Addison Run and
Bear Branch Loops

▓ **Quiet Hours:** 11 p.m.–7 a.m.

▓ **Visitors:** Must pay per-person fee
and be out by 10 p.m.

▓ **Fires:** In fire rings

▓ **Alcohol:** Permitted only inside
cabins and at shelters with valid
permit, as applicable

▓ **Stay Limit:** 2 weeks and can return
after 1 week

▓ **Other:** Checkout 1 p.m.

vistas, including Chimney Rock and Wolf Rock. While you're at it, try the Old Misery Trail—if nothing else, you've got to love the (somewhat misleading) name.

Sites in Cunningham Falls State Park are wooded and large. There is also a camp store near the entrance road next to the Addison Run Loop, which has 25 sites. Addison Run is one of five loops here. The others are Bear Branch (sites 26–57), Catoctin Creek (58–89), Deer Spring Branch (89–117), and Elderberry (118–149). Of these, the electric sites are concentrated in the Addison Run Loop (though there are some electric sites in the other loops: site 44 in Bear Branch; site 79 in Catoctin Creek; sites 98, 113,

115, and 117 in Deer Spring Branch; and site 130 in Elderberry). Each loop has its own bathhouse. With all of this activity, your chances for solitude and privacy aren't great, but you can increase them by heading to Elderberry, which is the westernmost loop and farthest from the concentrated electric sites. In Elder-berry, I'd recommend sites 118–128 as well as 131 and 133. These seem to be the farthest from other sites, and each backs to the woods without any other camping behind. However, the best of the best, if privacy is what you're after, are 102, 104, 105, and 107 in Deer Spring Branch Loop; all of them back up to woods and are comparatively private.

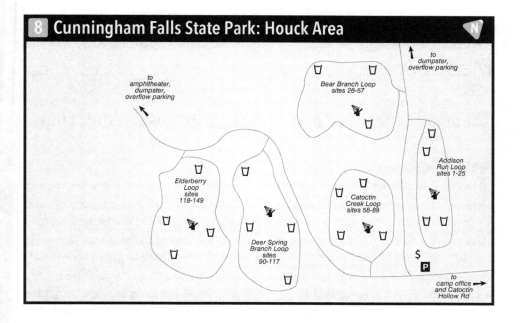

If you've brought the kids, don't miss the Catoctin Wildlife Preserve and Zoo, just across US 15 in Thurmont. With more than 400 animals—from rare monkeys and birds to jaguars, lions, and tigers— it's a great place to spend a few hours.

:: Getting There

Take I-70 to Frederick, and then US 15 north to Thurmont. Follow MD 77 west 4 miles to Catoctin Hollow Road.

GPS COORDINATES   N39°37'53" W77°28'16"

9

Cunningham Falls State Park:
Manor Area

The area has returned once more to an almost-pristine state.

The first settlers arrived at the foot of the Catoctin Mountains, in the Monocacy River valley, around 1730. The area's abundance of natural resources meant that industry wouldn't be too far behind. The starkest reminder of that time is the Catoctin Iron Furnace. In use from 1776 until the beginning of the 20th century, the furnace cast raw iron and iron tools. It once churned out ammunition for the Continental Army during the Revolutionary War. One of the brothers who founded the furnace would become governor of Maryland soon after. The furnace ran on charcoal, and the surrounding forests were slowly denuded to provide the requisite fuel. Fortunately, it's been more than a century since the practice stopped, and the area, now Cunningham Falls State Park, has returned once more to an almost-pristine state. The furnace is situated close to the Manor camping area and remains a relatively easy and popular hike from the end of the picnic area. Also nearby (running right through the camping area) is Little Hunting Creek, which provides put-and-take trout fishing.

The Manor Camping Area has 31 sites total. There are only one-fifth the number of sites of the William Houck Area here, and many people regard the Manor Area as a second choice if they can't get a place in William Houck. As a result, unless it's high season and a weekend, you may have a good chunk of the camping area to yourself.

So why do people prefer the more crowded Houck area? Perhaps it's because the Manor area sits not far off US 15; by contrast, Houck is several miles within park boundaries. This proximity to US 15 is off-putting to some people, but I've never heard road noise at Manor. The area is sufficiently forested, and US 15 is not a heavily traveled road, especially at night, so I wouldn't count this proximity as a detraction. However, those seeking complete solitude should at least note the location.

:: Ratings

BEAUTY: ★ ★ ★ ★
PRIVACY: ★ ★ ★
SPACIOUSNESS: ★ ★ ★
QUIET: ★ ★ ★ ★
SECURITY: ★ ★ ★ ★ ★
CLEANLINESS: ★ ★ ★ ★ ★

:: Key Information

ADDRESS: Cunningham Falls State Park
14039 Catoctin Hollow Road
Thurmont, MD 21788

CONTACT: 301-271-7574;
dnr2.maryland.gov

OPERATED BY: Maryland Department
of Natural Resources

OPEN: Early April–late October;
open without showers late October–
mid-December

SITES: 31

EACH SITE: Dust pad, picnic table, fire
ring, lantern post

ASSIGNMENT: First come, first served
April–Memorial Day and Labor Day–
end of the season; reservations recommended otherwise

REGISTRATION: 888-432-CAMP
(2267), **reservations.dnr.state.md.us,**
or at campground registration off
Catoctin Hollow Road

FACILITIES: Bathhouse, playground,
picnic area

PARKING: In designated sites

FEE: $21.49 plus service charge/night;
$27.49 plus service charge/night elec-
tric; additional day-use service charge
during high season $3–$5

RESTRICTIONS

▨ **Pets:** Allowed

▨ **Quiet Hours:** 11 p.m.–7 a.m.

▨ **Visitors:** Must pay per-person fee
and be out by 10 p.m.

▨ **Fires:** In fire rings

▨ **Alcohol:** Permitted only inside
cabins and at shelters with valid
permit, as applicable

▨ **Stay Limit:** 2 weeks, can return after
2 weeks

▨ **Other:** Checkout 1 p.m.

Electric sites in the Manor area are 6, 7, 9, 10, 15, and 17–21. They are cleverly lined along internal camp roads, which means that the outer sites, away from those internal roads, remain quieter. The most private of these outer sites are 1–3, 13, and 23–29. That said, two of my favorite sites in the park, notable for their relative privacy, are internal: 12 and 14.

From the Manor area, you can easily reach the park's other attractions by taking the Catoctin Trail, a 27-mile trail that runs from south of Frederick in Gambrill State Park, through Frederick, and into Cunningham Falls State Park; the portion of the trail within the park boundaries runs just under 9 miles. The trail also functions as a popular spur of the Appalachian Trail, which is merely 2 miles away where Raven Rock Road (MD 491) and Fort Ritchie Road intersect.

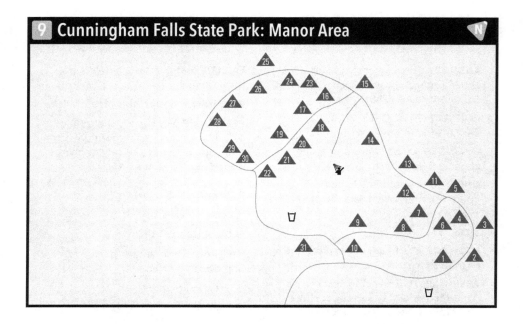

9 Cunningham Falls State Park: Manor Area

:: Getting There

From Frederick, take US 15 north toward Thurmont. The Manor area is 3 miles south of Thurmont directly off US 15.

GPS COORDINATES N39°37'53" W77°28'16"

10

Deep Creek Lake State Park

Many Marylanders might be surprised to know that this portion of their state actually lies west of the Eastern Continental Divide.

The obvious main attraction here is the proximity to Deep Creek Lake, a 3,900-acre lake and a four-season recreation area that draws from several surrounding states. Because many Marylanders tend to think of our eastern waters when they think of this kind of recreation, it means Garrett County is actually more popular with those in Pennsylvania and Ohio than many eastern-minded Maryland residents. Additionally, what many Marylanders would be surprised to know is that this portion of their state actually lies west of the Eastern Continental Divide, meaning that rainfall and snowmelt flow to the Mississippi, not the Atlantic. In this sense, Deep Creek Lake State Park is the

:: Ratings

BEAUTY: ★ ★ ★ ★
PRIVACY: ★ ★ ★
SPACIOUSNESS: ★ ★ ★
QUIET: ★ ★
SECURITY: ★ ★ ★ ★ ★
CLEANLINESS: ★ ★ ★ ★ ★

best of both worlds: water and mountains. Abutting both Meadow Mountain and Deep Creek Lake, it offers even more of an attraction: while much of the real estate surrounding the lake has skyrocketed and pushed rental rates beyond the means of many working families, the state park's campgrounds offer a great alternative.

What surrounds the campground is what makes camping here worth it, even if you find the site too populated—and expect crowds, especially in high season. The vast majority of campers cross over State Park Road to head to the lake, which offers a paradise of boating, swimming, and fishing. Day-users generally congregate on and near the lake too.

But if you want to escape the crush, it's easy to do so. Don't expect to have the hiking trails all to yourself, but don't expect much traffic either. Deep Creek State Park contains some wonderful trails, all easily accessible from the campground. So while it seems everyone is heading south to the lake, you can go north and escape. (Do leave time for enjoying the lake, however.) Had you

:: Key Information

ADDRESS: Deep Creek Lake State Park
898 State Park Road
Swanton, MD 21561

CONTACT: 301-387-5563;
dnr2.maryland.gov

OPERATED BY: Maryland Department
of Natural Resources

OPEN: Mid-April–mid-December

SITES: 101 (plus cabins, shelters, and
a yurt)

EACH SITE: Grill, picnic table, lantern
post, tent pad, metal food storage
container

ASSIGNMENT: First come, first served
late April–late May and mid-October–
mid-December; reservations otherwise

REGISTRATION: 888-432-CAMP
(2267) or **reservations.dnr.state.md.us**

FACILITIES: Ball fields, bathhouses,
boat rental and launch, dumping station, concessions, swimming beach,
playgrounds, shelters

PARKING: 2 vehicles at site, off-site for
additional vehicles

FEE: $21.49 plus service charge/night,
$27.49 plus service charge/night elec-
tric; additional day-use service charge
during high season $3–$5

RESTRICTIONS

■ **Pets:** Allowed in Browning,
Beckman, and Garrett Loops

■ **Quiet Hours:** 11 p.m.–7 a.m.

■ **Visitors:** Maximum 6 people/site

■ **Fires:** In fire ring only

■ **Alcohol:** Permitted only inside
cabins and at shelters with valid
permit, as applicable

■ **Stay Limit:** 2 weeks

■ **Other:** This is bear country—take
proper precautions. For tips on how to
camp among bears, visit **dnr.state.md
.us/wildlife/HuntTrap/blackbear
/bblivingwith.asp.**

been hiking here a century ago, virgin red spruce, hemlock, white pine, and yellow birch would have been the dominant tree species, but massive logging operations cleared the land. Fortunately, the Department of Natural Resources estimates that more than 95 percent of the park has regenerated. Now the forest consists mostly of oak and hickory. Much fauna makes its home here, too, with black bears and bobcats perhaps the most glamorous. The campsites that offer the easiest access to the mountain trails are 34–40 in the Delphia Brant Loop and

60–67 between the George Beckman and John Garret Loops.

Because of its location in such a popular tourist area, Deep Creek State Park doesn't allow for much isolation. But for those looking not for a backcountry experience but for a wonderful time full of activities, the park is perfect. Its Discover Center offers hands-on exhibits and programs highlighting the area's natural and cultural heritage. Park rangers and naturalists regularly schedule hikes and evening campfire programs that are always fun and informative.

After entering on State Park Road and passing the camp headquarters, you'll immediately come to two loops: one to the left (Meshach Browning Loop) and one to the right (Delphia Brant Loop). You're best avoiding the Browning Loop, as this is where the electric sites are congregated. (Of the other sites in the park, some are tent-only and others can accommodate RVs but do not have electrical hookups.) Meshach Browning has sites 1–26, while Delphia Brant contains sites 27–52. Five more sites sit along a spur loop just north of site 40, which leads to cabins and a yurt. The first impression of the campground isn't the best one, especially if it's high season. The initial sites are close together and chockablock with RVs. But don't despair; keep heading away from these first loops. (If you do wind up in either of these loops, try for site 40, which sits on a nicely wooded corner; to the right of it is the spur loop with sites 52–57, dead-end sites with nothing behind them. These aren't bad at all.)

Beyond the first loops are the better options: George Beckman and John Garrett Loops, where you'll find sites 58–112. Each loop contains its own bathhouse and doesn't differ significantly from the other. But the farther away you go from the entrance, the quieter it seems to get and the more spacious the sites. You'll have more privacy here. Site 69 and the sites in the low 70s are nice, sitting on the farthest edge of the campground. My favorite of these is site 64; it sits behind a big rock ridge and has a trail heading up the hill behind it. The sites in these loops are nice, and you should be quite happy with them. I would recommend avoiding only the sites right next to the bathhouse: 81, 95, 97, and 107.

In short, the campsites are reasonably shaded and roomy, each measuring roughly 24 by 24 feet. Still, this is your garden-variety campground—full of basic amenities and with decent tree buffers, but usually crowded. What can't be disputed is that it remains a wonderful alternative to pricier options in this resort area.

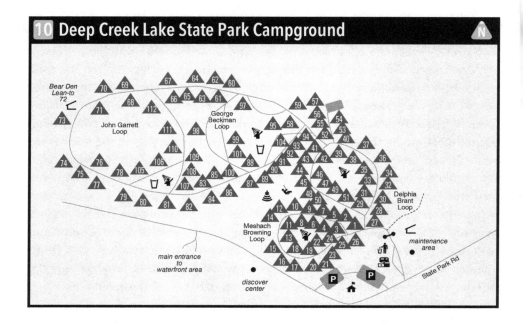

:: Getting There

Take I-68 to Exit 14A (MD 219 South to Deep Creek Lake). Continue on MD 219 South for 18 miles. Turn left onto Glendale Road. Continue on Glendale Road for 1 mile. Immediately after crossing Glendale Bridge, turn left onto State Park Road.

GPS COORDINATES   N39°30'34" W79°23'28"

11

Fort Frederick State Park

Fort Frederick is the country's best-preserved French and Indian stone fort.

Fort Frederick is perhaps the best place to view the span of Maryland's military history: During the French and Indian War, it served as a defense fortification; during the Revolutionary War, as a prison; and during the Civil War, as a defense of the Chesapeake & Ohio Canal. It proved to be impenetrable, owing to its thick stone wall construction (as opposed to most forts of the era, which were constructed of wood or earth). Year-round military reenactments, interpretive guides, and a historical center in the fort complex allow for fascinating access to the country's best-preserved French and Indian stone fort. Restorations begun in the 1920s by the Civilian Conservation Corps continued all the way through the fort's 250th birthday, which was celebrated in 2006.

:: Ratings

BEAUTY: ★ ★ ★ ★
PRIVACY: ★ ★
SPACIOUSNESS: ★ ★
QUIET: ★ ★ ★ ★
SECURITY: ★ ★ ★ ★ ★
CLEANLINESS: ★ ★ ★ ★ ★

The fort's location makes it a prime attraction. Parkland contains sections of the Potomac River, C&O Canal, Big Pool, and the Western Maryland Rail Trail (WMRT), a 23-mile paved path that follows the former Western Maryland Railway line. The Rails-to-Trails Conservancy has recognized the WMRT as one of the country's best trails for viewing fall foliage. Of course, there's also the C&O Canal Towpath, which follows the Potomac some 185 miles from Washington, D.C., to Cumberland, Maryland. (For camping along the C&O, see pages 21–36).

The Potomac allows for great swimming (be careful; the currents can be deceptively swift midriver), boating, and fishing. The species of fish, both native and introduced, number in the dozens—bass, carp, catfish, crappie, eel, herring, perch, pickerel, shad, sunfish, and trout among them.

One couldn't ask for a better location for a campground. Fort Frederick sits up the hill, easily accessible via a paved path (Fort Frederick Road). Down from the fort, you cross the C&O Canal Towpath running alongside Big Pool. The campground sits between the towpath and the

:: Key Information

ADDRESS: Fort Frederick State Park
11100 Fort Frederick Road
Big Pool, MD 21711

CONTACT: 301-842-2155;
dnr2.maryland.gov

OPERATED BY: Maryland Department of Natural Resources

OPEN: Early April–early November

SITES: 29

EACH SITE: Grill, lantern hook, picnic table, tent pad, fire ring

ASSIGNMENT: Reservations required for wheelchair-accessible sites; otherwise, register at park or in advance

REGISTRATION: first come, first served or at **reservations.dnr.state.md.us**

FACILITIES: Boat launch, camp store, picnic, playground, shelters, visitor center

PARKING: On gravel driveway, maximum 2 vehicles/site

FEE: $15/night, $16/night out-of-state residents; includes park entrance fee

RESTRICTIONS

■ **Pets:** Allowed on leash and attended

■ **Quiet Hours:** 11 p.m.–7 a.m.

■ **Visitors:** Maximum 6 people/site

■ **Fires:** In fire rings

■ **Alcohol:** Permitted only inside cabins and at shelters with valid permit, as applicable

■ **Stay Limit:** 2 weeks

■ **Other:** Checkout 3 p.m.

Potomac River. There are only 29 sites total; 1–17 are arguably the best, as they sit waterside (the Potomac), while 18–29 sit on the other side of the campground road, nearer Big Pool and the C&O Canal Towpath (not a bad location either). Depending on one's particular wants and needs, note that a restroom sits closest to site 1 and that steps down to the river are closest to site 8. Sites 19 and 20, second- and third-farthest down the campground road, are wheelchair accessible and share a restroom between them. These sites require reservations.

The campground itself is basically one open space, with the sites sitting right next to each other, with 25 feet (and no trees) between them. Thus, there's little in the way of privacy. The entire campground is a few hundred yards at best. However, as the sites sit either right alongside the river or just across the path, there really is no bad spot if you can get over the lack of privacy. Plus, the area is incredibly beautiful. *Note:* Train tracks lie on the far side of the river (in West Virginia), so you may hear trains now and again.

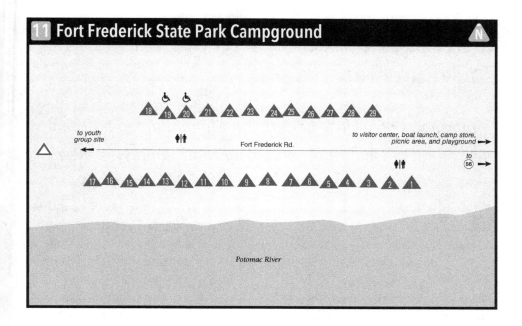

11 Fort Frederick State Park Campground

to youth group site

to visitor center, boat launch, camp store, picnic area, and playground

Fort Frederick Rd.

to 56

Potomac River

:: Getting There

Take I-70 to Exit 12 (Big Pool/Indian Springs, MD 56). Turn east on Big Pool Road, and the park entrance will be 1.2 miles on the left.

GPS COORDINATES N39°36'36" W78°0'12"

12

Gambrill State Park:
Rock Run Area

Gambrill sits on a ridge of Catoctin Mountain and contains the summit of High Knob, providing some impressive views.

Gambrill State Park, at more than 1,100 acres, is located within an area of Frederick County that's packed with recreation opportunities. Gambrill sits on a ridge of Catoctin Mountain and contains the summit of High Knob, modest at 1,600 feet but providing some impressive views: Frederick City Municipal Forest to the north, Gathland State Park and the Middletown and Monocacy Valleys to the south, and the Civil War historical site—South Mountain—to the west.

Gambrill State Park is divided into two recreational areas: Rock Run, at the park entrance, is where you'll find the campground; High Knob encompasses the top of Catoctin Mountain.

:: Ratings

BEAUTY: ★ ★ ★ ★
PRIVACY: ★ ★ ★
SPACIOUSNESS: ★ ★
QUIET: ★ ★ ★
SECURITY: ★ ★ ★ ★ ★
CLEANLINESS: ★ ★ ★ ★

Midway between the two areas is the Trailhead Parking Lot, which provides access to Gambrill's 16 miles of hiking trails, including access to the Catoctin Trail, a 27-mile trail that traverses Gambrill, Catoctin Mountain Park, Cunningham Falls State Park, and Frederick City Municipal Forest.

The campground at Rock Run sits south of the trails. Because the sites are nicely wooded and relatively minimal in number, the campground rarely feels crowded. It's true that you're never too far from neighbors, but also there will never be too many of them. When I camp here, it usually feels relatively empty, though there never seem to be too many vacant sites. The pace is relaxed. There's also a small pond in Rock Run, stocked with bass, bluegill, and catfish.

There are 34 sites in all, including four full-service cabins, numbered 4, 5, 6, and 18. After the electric sites (1, 12, 13, 20, 22), a relatively small number of sites are left for tent campers. Of these, only sites 23–27 and 30–34 are tent-only. Sites 30–34 sit on the farthest section from the entrance, up

:: Key Information

ADDRESS: Gambrill State Park
8602 Gambrill Park Road
Frederick, MD 21702

CONTACT: 301-271-7574;
dnr2.maryland.gov

OPERATED BY: Maryland Department
of Natural Resources

OPEN: Early April–late October

SITES: 30 (plus 4 camper cabins)

EACH SITE: Grill, lantern hook, picnic
table, tent pad

ASSIGNMENT: First come, first served
early April–late May and September–
end of the season; reservations always
available

REGISTRATION: For self-registration,
pick available site and register within
30 minutes. For reservations,
call 888-432-CAMP (2267) or go to
reservations.dnr.state.md.us.

FACILITIES: Bathhouses, picnic shelters, playground

PARKING: All vehicles must be on
gravel drive, except in tent-only sites

FEE: $18.49 plus service charge/night,
$24.49 plus service charge/night elec-
tric; additional day-use service charge
during high season $3–$5

RESTRICTIONS

▓ **Pets:** On a leash and attended

▓ **Quiet Hours:** 11 p.m.–7 a.m.

▓ **Visitors:** Maximum 8 people/site

▓ **Fires:** In fire ring

▓ **Alcohol:** Permitted only inside
cabins and at shelters with valid
permit, as applicable

▓ **Stay Limit:** 2 weeks

▓ **Other:** Checkout 3 p.m.

the hill; however, they also sit near a camp road and are far from spectacular. That said, a bonus to sites 30–34 is that they sit right in front of the red trail, which you'd take to access all the other park trails. Of these sites, I like the rocks and mature trees that decorate site 31. In general, the higher up the hill you go, the nicer the sites are. The sites in the first tent-only area, 23–27, are in a middle section with roads nearby and are very close to one another.

Of course, you're not limited to the tent-only sites, even if you only have a tent. The rule of thumb, again, is to keep heading away from the entrance. This means that the first ones you come to, 1–7 and 19–27, are best avoided. Heading away from the entrance, sites 8–18 and 30–34 are your best bets. If, however, you desire easy access to a swing set and an open field, where kids might kick a ball or throw a Frisbee, go for sites 9, 10, or 11.

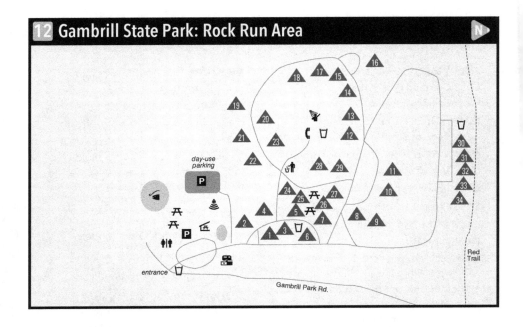

:: Getting There

From Frederick, follow US 15 to US 40 W (pass US Alternate 40) and exit to Gambrill Park Road.

GPS COORDINATES   N39°28'43" W77°29'29"

13

Garrett State Forest:
Snaggy Mountain Area

The sites are all spacious, private, and located in a stunning natural setting.

A word of warning: The Garrett State Forest's camping areas aren't easy to locate because they're sandwiched between two prominent state parks: Swallow Falls and Herrington Manor. In fact, it's more accurate to say that the two state parks are located within the forest, and the forest is easily mistaken as a greenbelt between Swallow Falls and Herrington Manor. Both state parks have well-established camping facilities (Herrington Manor is cabin-only), and, as a result, people are often unaware that they can camp in the forest as well. The largest and best-maintained camping section in the forest sits between the two parks and is called the Snaggy Mountain Area. It's a

wonderful—if underutilized—primitive camping area.

The Garrett State Forest is where forestry conservation in Maryland began. The Garrett Brothers owned the western forestlands in this area; in 1906, they donated more than 1,900 acres to the state. Today, the holdings that constitute the state forest total more than 7,000 acres. It's an area of rugged and wooded mountain terrain, speckled with streams and rivers and home to an abundance of wildlife, including many black bears.

The camping area sits off unpaved Snaggy Mountain Road (see directions below). Note that the northern entrance is closed to through traffic, so you'll need to make your entrance on the south side, where the self-registration kiosk is located. Taking in portions of Snaggy Mountain Road is the Garrett Trail, a 7-mile hike that offers stunning sights in the forest: river valleys, hemlock groves, and wetlands. The trail also passes (and sometimes encompasses) two other prominent trails: Backbone Mountain and Potomac River. Additionally, a

:: Ratings

BEAUTY: ★ ★ ★ ★ ★
PRIVACY: ★ ★ ★ ★ ★
QUIET: ★ ★ ★ ★ ★
SPACIOUSNESS: ★ ★ ★ ★ ★
SECURITY: ★ ★ ★
CLEANLINESS: ★ ★ ★ ★ ★

:: Key Information

ADDRESS: Potomac-Garrett SF
1431 Potomac Camp Road
Oakland, MD 21550

CONTACT: 301-334-2038;
dnr2.maryland.gov

OPERATED BY: Maryland Department
of Natural Resources

OPEN: Year-round, but roads are not
maintained in winter

SITES: 11

EACH SITE: Lantern hook, grill, picnic
table

ASSIGNMENT: First come, first served

REGISTRATION: Self-registration
station on Snaggy Mountain Road;
call Forest office for reservations at
301-334-2038

FACILITIES: None

PARKING: Vehicles must be parked on
gravel portion of site

FEE: $10/night

RESTRICTIONS

▨ **Pets:** Permitted

▨ **Quiet Hours:** 11 p.m.–7 a.m.

▨ **Visitors:** Maximum 8 people or
2 units/site

▨ **Fires:** In fire rings only

▨ **Alcohol:** Permitted only inside
cabins and at shelters with valid
permit, as applicable

▨ **Stay Limit:** 2 weeks

▨ **Other:** Checkout 3 p.m. This is bear
country–take proper precautions. For
tips on how to camp among bears,
visit **dnr.state.md.us/wildlife/Hunt
Trap/blackbear/bblivingwith.asp.**

5.5-mile trail runs through the area and connects the two state parks. At Herrington Manor, a 53-acre lake anchors a popular recreation area. (For a description of Swallow Falls, see pages 100–102.)

In short, there's a plethora of hiking opportunities in the Snaggy Mountain Area, all of them within a short jaunt from the campsites. Be aware, however, that most forest trails are open not only to hikers but also to skiers, equestrians, snowmobilers, and off-road vehicle operators. (The exception to this is the Herrington Manor's Swallow Falls Trail, which doesn't allow motorized vehicles.) Still, don't let this dissuade you from camping here;

it's truly a beautiful spot. I would recommend, however, getting hold of a trail map from the Garrett State Forest headquarters (see above for contact info) before setting out. Similar to the Potomac State Forest, which is maintained by the same section of the Department of Natural Resources, the sites are all spacious, private, and located in a stunning natural setting. They also often sit a quarter of a mile or more from one another. And, just like in the Potomac State Forest, you can't go wrong with any one of them. In fact, I would recommend simply taking the first available site (if nothing else, it saves the jarring on your car). But if you are inclined

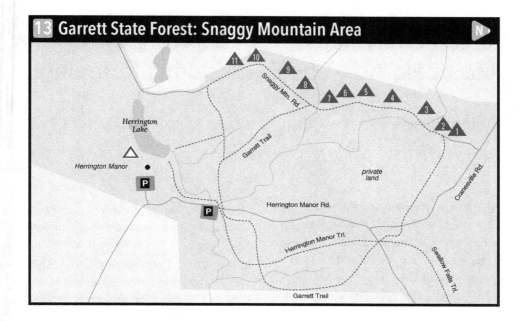

13 Garrett State Forest: Snaggy Mountain Area

to take the whole of Snaggy Mountain Road toward the northern reaches, site 2 is one of the most gorgeous camping spots I've seen. Covered in pine needles, it sits in a grove of hemlocks and has an abundance of level ground for tents.

All 11 sites sit along Snaggy Mountain Road, but passing vehicles will be few and slow-moving, as the roads are unpaved and very bumpy. Again, simply choose the first available site; you can't go wrong.

:: Getting There

From Deep Creek Lake, take MD 219 south for 2 miles to a right on Mayhew Inn Road and go 4.5 miles to a stop sign. Turn left onto Oakland Sang Run Road, and then take the first right onto Swallow Falls Road. Pass Swallow Falls State Park and take a left onto Herrington Manor Road. Drive 4.4 miles and turn right onto Tomar Drive. Go half a mile and turn right onto Fingerboard Road. Travel 1.7 miles and turn right onto Sanders Lane to the Snaggy Mountain Road South entrance.

GPS COORDINATES   N39°29'46.9"   W79°27'18.2"

14

Garrett State Forest: Piney
Mountain Area and Backcountry Camping

Camping here is a real out-of-the-way experience, and it's well worth the trouble locating it.

In the description of Garrett State Forest: Snaggy Mountain Area on pages 53–55, I mention that the forest camping area can be difficult to locate. In the case of the Piney Mountain Area of the forest, that goes double. It seems easy enough, but the northern portion of the state forest (where the Piney Mountain Area is located) is a patchwork of non-contiguous public lands surrounded by private holdings. Further, because of the rural nature of the area, there are few markers to guide you.

However, the problems listed above are a by-product of the fact that camping here is a real out-of-the-way experience, and it's well worth the necessary trouble locating it. The six sites within the Piney Mountain Area constitute huge, cleared areas carved from the forest that sit along the unpaved Piney Mountain Road. They are essentially identical to the sites in the Snaggy Mountain Area. The real difference between the two is that Piney Mountain is more remote and doesn't see nearly the same amount of through-traffic created by Snaggy Mountain's much closer proximity to Herrington Manor and Swallow Falls State Parks (though, to be fair, "traffic" here is a relative term). Also, camping at Piney Mountain offers easy access to one of Maryland's natural oddities. Straddling the Maryland–West Virginia border on Cranesville Road just to the west of the Piney Mountain Area is the Cranesville Swamp. This is a subarctic swamp, hosting a landscape that one rarely ever finds south of Canada. A perfect storm of environmental conditions created it, and it hosts birds and flowers that otherwise can't be seen this far south.

Piney Mountain Road is an unpaved forest road that leads to a secondary loop trail where motorized vehicles are

:: Ratings

BEAUTY ★ ★ ★ ★ ★
PRIVACY ★ ★ ★ ★ ★
QUIET ★ ★ ★ ★ ★
SPACIOUSNESS ★ ★ ★ ★ ★
SECURITY ★ ★
CLEANLINESS ★ ★ ★ ★ ★

:: Key Information

ADDRESS: Potomac-Garrett SF
1431 Potomac Camp Road
Oakland, MD 21550

CONTACT: 301-334-2038;
dnr2.maryland.gov

OPERATED BY: Maryland Department
of Natural Resources

OPEN: Year-round, but roads are not
maintained in winter

SITES: 6+ (6 in Piney Mountain Area,
unlimited in forest backcountry)

EACH SITE: Lantern hook, grill, picnic
table (Piney Mountain Area)

ASSIGNMENT: First come, first served

REGISTRATION: Self-registration
station on Piney Mountain Road

FACILITIES: None

PARKING: Vehicles must be parked
on gravel portion of site, off road in
forest

FEE: $10/night

RESTRICTIONS

▧ **Pets:** Permitted

▧ **Quiet Hours:** 11 a.m.–7 p.m.

▧ **Visitors:** Maximum 8 people or 2
units

▧ **Fires:** In fire rings only

▧ **Alcohol:** Permitted only inside
cabins and at shelters with valid
permit, as applicable

▧ **Stay Limit:** 2 weeks

▧ **Other:** Check-in and checkout
3 p.m. for roadside sites. Camping
prohibited within 200 feet of any trail
or stream. This is bear country—take
proper precautions. For tips on how to
camp among bears, visit **dnr.state
.md.us/wildlife/HuntTrap/blackbear
/bblivingwith.asp.**

prohibited. The campsites sit along the road and are hardly distinguishable from one another—in a good way. They are all spacious, far from the next site, and sit within pristine forest. Like the other sites in Garrett Forest (and Potomac State Forest), you can't go wrong with any one of them. Take the first one that is available; you'll be quite happy with it. Aside from the privacy and out-of-the-way feel of the campsites in Piney Mountain, its general proximity to the two state parks listed above means it's a less expensive, more private alternative, albeit without the facilities one would enjoy at a state park.

If the idea of a fire grill, lantern hook, and picnic table means that, in your view, you're not at all roughing it, you can also camp anywhere in the forest where there are not established sites, provided you have obtained a backcountry permit. For Piney Mountain, this effectively means the area south of Sang Run Road and between Piney Mountain Road and Cranesville Road. For the Snaggy Mountain Area (see pages 53–55), this backcountry experience can be enjoyed in the large swath of forest between Herrington Manor and Swallow Falls, with the exception of a large, privately held area, marked accordingly.

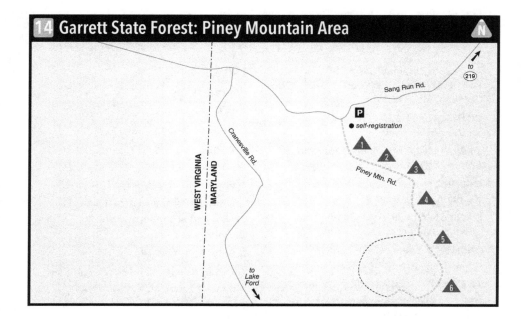

14 Garrett State Forest: Piney Mountain Area

:: Getting There

From I-68, take Exit 14 and travel south on MD 219 for roughly 15 miles to a right on Sang Run Road. Follow to a left onto Piney Mountain Road (if you reach Cranesville Road, turn around and look for Piney Mountain to the right).

GPS COORDINATES   N39°32'56.5" W79°27'43.5"

15

Green Ridge State Forest

These are wonderful campsites, all far from one another, within pristine forested settings, and with plenty of space to pitch several tents.

Want to get away from it all? Camping in Green Ridge State Forest is almost too good to be true: 100 primitive campsites within 44,000 acres of oak and hickory forest.

After Savage River State Forest, Green Ridge is Maryland's second-largest state forest. The forest encompasses Green Ridge Mountain and Polish Mountain, as well as 2,039-foot Town Hill, the forest's highest point. It also happens to be my favorite camping destination in Maryland. This is because it's only two hours from my home in Baltimore, lacks the massive crowds heading east to the ocean and the better-known recreation areas to the west, and allows for truly spectacular,

:: Ratings

> BEAUTY: ★ ★ ★ ★ ★
> PRIVACY: ★ ★ ★ ★ ★
> SPACIOUSNESS: ★ ★ ★ ★ ★
> QUIET: ★ ★ ★ ★ ★
> SECURITY: ★ ★ ★
> CLEANLINESS: ★ ★ ★ ★ ★

away-from-it-all camping. At $10 a night, it's also an absolute bargain.

I've broken up the widely dispersed campsites for Green Ridge State Forest into three areas. It makes sense to focus on one of the three areas per trip, but do make subsequent trips to explore the other areas. Aside from the fact that the unpaved roads and size of the forest can make getting from campsite to campsite a long and arduous process, breaking the sites up the way I have done (north of I-68 [sites 1–23], west of Green Ridge [24–52], and east of Green Ridge [53–100]) means that you can choose your campsite based on one of three options: If you desire a quick and easy escape, go for the sites north of I-68; if you want forested bliss and access to the western hiking trails, go for the west side of Green Ridge; and if you desire forest but wish for easier access to the C&O Canal and the Potomac River, go for the east side of Green Ridge. If you want to choose your stay based on certain activities, here's a rough guide: Choose sites 1–54 for hunting; 24–49, 55–79, and 86–88 for equestrian use; 80–85 and

:: Key Information

ADDRESS: Green Ridge State Forest 28700 Headquarters Drive NE Flintstone, MD 21530-9525

CONTACT: 301-478-3124; dnr2.maryland.gov

OPERATED BY: Maryland Department of Natural Resources

OPEN: Year-round

SITES: 100 (plus 7 group sites for 20+ people)

EACH SITE: Fire ring, picnic table

ASSIGNMENT: First come, first served

REGISTRATION: At the Green Ridge Visitor Center (see directions); use self-registration if the center is closed.

FACILITIES: Bathrooms, water at visitor center

PARKING: On gravel pad, off forest road

FEE: $10/night for up to 6 people, $1 each additional person

RESTRICTIONS

▓ **Pets:** Permitted on a leash

▓ **Quiet Hours:** None posted

▓ **Visitors:** See "Fee" above

▓ **Fires:** Permitted at sites but must be monitored at all times

▓ **Alcohol:** Permitted only inside cabins and at shelters with valid permit, as applicable

▓ **Stay Limit:** None; when you register, mark the intended length of stay

▓ **Other:** Must be at least 18 years of age to register for a site

90–100 for boating and fishing. No site is terribly far from a hiking trail (more than 50 miles in all in the forest), and forest roads are, in essence, "hikable" traverses.

Because the campsites are spread out across the forest, a good map is essential. But here's a rough guide for the sites north of I-68: Sites 1–23 sit nestled within the following approximate boundaries: I-68 to the south, Fifteen Mile Creek (and Fifteen Mile Creek Road) to the east, Old Cumberland Road to the north, and Treasure Road and Frank Davis Road to the west. It's evident that you'll be near a road, no matter what. But these are narrow, unpaved forest roads that don't see much traffic. It is reasonable, however, to want to be far away from I-68, which sees trucks throughout the night, but you might be surprised by how quiet this area

is despite its proximity to the interstate. The only two sites where you might hear regular road noise are those closest: site 1 on Fifteen Mile Creek Road and site 19 on Big Ridge Road. Site 1 is certainly the most convenient and will spare you the jarring of the roads, but my suggestion is to continue north along Fifteen Mile Creek Road and take the next left onto Carpenter Road. The first site you'll come to is site 11, on the right. This fantastic site is large and deep in the woods. Plus, you can easily walk back to Fifteen Mile and pick up the blue trail just behind. It is labeled Pine Lick Trail, and its terminus at the Mason-Dixon Line links with the 176-mile Mid-State Pennsylvania Trail.

Sites 12–15 are found continuing west along Carpenter. (If you have a large group, take site 12—it's enormous.)

Sites 2–4 are north up Fifteen Mile Creek Road. Just beyond Carpenter Road north is Double Pine Road, where you'll find sites 5–10, as well as a shelter site, convenient in case of bad weather. This site is off the little path just south of site 10. The rest in this section: Use Old Cumberland Road for site 4 (left from Fifteen Mile). Use Davis Road for sites 20–22 (left off Carpenter after the intersection with Treasure Road, which you would use to get to site 23, one of the most remote sites in all the forest). Last, use Big Ridge Road for sites 16–19 (the second left off Fifteen Mile just after exiting I-68).

To reach these sites, use Exit 62 (US 40/Fifteen Mile Creek Road) off I-68. All of the sites sit right off the forest road, so they're easy to find. Plus, the relentless pitch and yaw of your car on these roads means you'll probably want to simply find a suitable site and stop. When you find the site you want, you can call the visitor center (where you need to stop first and pay) and tell them where you are.

The state forest is best enjoyed west of Green Ridge, in the rising valley lands between Town Hill to the east and Polish Mountain to the west. Aside from some great hiking, there's also the forest's prime designated mountain-bike trail, 12 miles of up and down through some stunning scenery. Sites 24–52 lie southwest of I-68 and west of Green Ridge, the natural dividing line in the forest. Most of the activity in this section is centered near Wallizer Road, where there's mountain-bike trail parking, horseback riding, and fishing at White Sulphur Pond. Sites 29–32, as well as a group site (G1), sit near the pond along Wallizer. The main artery in this section is Green Ridge Road, which runs perpendicular to Wallizer. Sites 33 and 34 are also accessed using Green Ridge Road. Use Sugar Bottom Road for sites 24–28—these sites are also near the activities listed above but are not as close as those on Wallizer. If you prefer to stay far away from the action, head west, using Jacobs Road, for sites 41 and 49; Twigg Road for sites 38–40 and 44–48; May Road for 42 and 43; Gordon Road for 36 and 37; and Mertens Avenue for 35 and 38–40. Be aware that site 35 on Mertens Avenue sits just across the road from a group site (G2) but is also within easy walking distance of a great overlook south on Green Ridge Road.

Heading south along Fifteen Mile Creek Road from I-68, your second right is Sugar Bottom Road. Fifteen Mile then begins to zigzag before straightening out at Green Ridge Road (you have to veer right to get onto Green Ridge; if you pass site 55 to the left, you've gone too far). Now on Green Ridge, Wallizer is your next right; sites G1 and 32 are the first you come to, each close to White Sulphur Pond. Sites 33 and 34 are next along Green Ridge, then Mertens Avenue appears on the right. The first right off Mertens is Gordon Road (36 and 37, closest to the bike trails). Where you would turn right for Gordon, going left instead takes you past sites 38–40 and then to Twigg Road (left, sites 44–48) and May Road (right, site 42), and finally Jacobs Road (head right for site 41, left for 49–52). These last three sites are quite far, requiring a bumpy ride. An easier way to access sites 50–52 is by continuing on

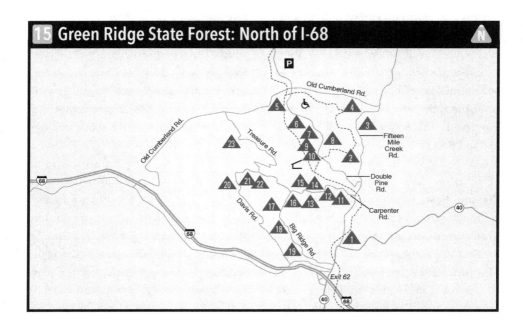

15 Green Ridge State Forest: North of I-68

Green Ridge South and taking a right on Jacobs. This will also take you past the fantastic Warrior Mountain Overlook, named for The Great Warrior Path, an American Indian trail linking the Carolinas to the Great Lakes. To access these sites, take Exit 62, Fifteen Mile Creek Road South.

The eastern section of the forest is characterized by its drop (losing about 700-plus feet of altitude) as it heads toward the Potomac River; here you'll find Green Ridge State Forest's most well-maintained infrastructure. Heading south along Green Ridge Road from the I-68 exit at Fifteen Mile Creek Road, you'll first pass the left turn to sites 55 and 56 just after the road stops its switchbacks. It's then a long ride (more than 2 miles) to a left on Mertens Road, heading east. You'll first come to sites 53 and 54. Continuing east on Mertens, you'll cross Stafford Road

(home of sites 57–63, which you'll reach in descending numerical order if you go north). If you go right down Stafford, you'll come to site 100, which sits by itself where Stafford and East Valley Road meet, not far from fishing at Orchard Pond. The good news is that these sites once sat next to an off-road vehicle trail that has been permanently closed. You can now use these sites without fear of loud engines.

If you keep heading east on Mertens, you'll pass group site G7, and next up is Oldtown Orleans Road, containing site 64 just to the south and 67–69 to the north, as well as group site G4. If you continue on Mertens, you'll come to some of my favorite sites, 65 and 66, which you'll reach by going right on Outdoor Club Road. This is a dead end, so there's no through-traffic, and these are the only two sites along its route. They sit atop the C&O Canal just in

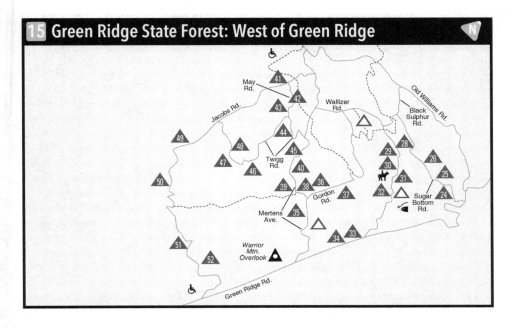

Green Ridge State Forest: West of Green Ridge

front of a beautiful sweep of the Potomac River, easily accessed.

If you don't continue on Mertens but instead keep heading north on Oldtown Orleans, past G4 and 67–69, you'll eventually hit sites 70–79. After site 79, you'll find yourself looping back toward sites 57–55 and Green Ridge Road, not far from where you came off I-68. Of these sites, I'd recommend site 74, which sits by itself on Howard Road, a right turn off Oldtown Orleans. After site 70 on Oldtown Orleans Road, heading south, you can take a left to reach Carroll Road. By going right on Carroll, you'll find sites 86–89, as well as G6 (between 87 and 88).

For the rest of the sites in this section, I recommend exiting I-68 at Exit 68 (Orleans Road south). If you do that, in about 3 miles, you'll come to Mountain Road. Here, you'll find group site G5, plus 80–83 by going right on Mountain. Of these, I like 80 and 81 best, as they sit astride Fifteen Mile Creek. If you take a left on Yonkers Bottom Road between G5 and site 83, you'll reach site 84, a great remote spot on Fifteen Mile Creek. Site 85 is difficult to get to and may not be worth the effort if you go there and it's already taken, but it's an incredible site, completely on its own off Cliff Road above Sideling Hill Creek. To reach it, take the second left off Orleans Road (Price Road) and then a right on Hoop Pole Road to a right on Stottlemeyer Road. Look for it on the right.

Lastly, sites 90–99 should be your preference if you've brought the canoe or kayak, as they all lie near the Bonds Landing boat launch on Kasecamp Road. Sites 90–98 are the few sites in the forest that don't offer too much privacy. Of these, though, you might want to consider site

15 Green Ridge State Forest: East of Green Ridge

99, which offers the best bet for privacy, sitting by itself to the northeast along Kasecamp. To reach these sites, go as far east as you can on Mertens, and then take a U-turn right on Kasecamp. (Be aware: This is not an easy trip in any vehicle, and it's probably not worth the effort if you're trailing a boat.)

:: Getting There

To the visitor center: Take I-68 to Exit 64 south (M.V. Smith Road). Go a few hundred yards to a right at the visitor center.

GPS COORDINATES   Visitor Center: N39°39'55.3" W78°26'34.2"

16

Greenbrier State Park

Annapolis Rock has a well-deserved reputation as a place to while away hours simply sitting and taking it all in.

Greenbrier State Park, at just under 1,300 acres, has two main attractions: the Appalachian Trail and the 42-acre Greenbrier Lake. The lake provides good fishing, as it's stocked with trout, largemouth bass, and bluegill; a Maryland Angler's License is required for fishermen 16 years of age or older. It also serves as a great place for a swim, with its nice beach; lifeguards are on duty 11 a.m.–6 p.m.

Bartman's Hill Trail leaves from the visitor center and heads directly to the Appalachian Trail. While some 12 miles of trails run throughout the western reaches of the park, many people ignore them and give in to the cache of hiking the AT, even if just for a day or two. Once you reach the AT from Bartman's Hill Trail, it's 3 miles in either direction to two popular sites: Annapolis Rock to the north and Washington Monument State Park to the south.

:: Ratings

BEAUTY: ★ ★ ★ ★
PRIVACY: ★ ★
SPACIOUSNESS: ★ ★
QUIET: ★ ★ ★
SECURITY: ★ ★ ★ ★ ★
CLEANLINESS: ★ ★ ★ ★ ★

At 1,700 feet elevation, Annapolis Rock is fairly modest in height (even by Maryland standards), but the view it commands over Greenbrier Lake and the Cumberland Valley earns it a well-deserved reputation as a place to while away hours simply sitting and taking it all in.

Heading the other way, Washington Monument State Park is a small park at only 108 acres, but it contains a true piece of American history: the country's first monument to our first president. Within a couple of hours, you can see the most famous Washington Monument in D.C. and the most beautiful one in Mount Vernon, Baltimore, but the historic one that stands in Washington Monument State Park has as its chief attraction a rather touching austerity. It stands only 34 feet tall as a circular wall of dry rock.

As for the camping, there are four loops, each with a bathhouse. It's a pretty campground, with many of the sites following the natural contours of the land. It's also a heavily wooded campground, and maintenance is impeccable. The Ash Loop (A) is nearest the entrance and visitor center and contains 31 sites (site 2 is reserved for the camp host). A path heading to the lake sits to the south of

:: Key Information

ADDRESS: Greenbrier State Park
21843 National Pike
Boonsboro, MD 21713-9535

CONTACT: 301-791-4767;
dnr2.maryland.gov

OPERATED BY: Maryland Department
of Natural Resources

OPEN: Early April–late October

SITES: 165

EACH SITE: Picnic table, grill, lantern
hook, tent pad

ASSIGNMENT: Reservations required

REGISTRATION: 888-432-CAMP
(2267) or **reservations.dnr.state.md.us**

FACILITIES: Picnic tables, grills, playgrounds, swimming beach, boat
launch, boat rental, camp store,
bathhouses, dump station

PARKING: Vehicles must remain on
gravel driveway

FEE: $21.49 plus service charge/night,
$27.49 plus service charge/night elec-
tric; additional day-use service charge
during high season $3–$5

RESTRICTIONS

▓ **Pets:** Allowed in Cedar and
Dogwood loops

▓ **Quiet Hours:** 11 p.m.–7 a.m.

▓ **Visitors:** Maximum 6 people/site

▓ **Fires:** In fire rings

▓ **Alcohol:** Permitted only inside
cabins and at shelters with valid
permit, as applicable

▓ **Stay Limit:** 2 weeks

▓ **Other:** Checkout 3 p.m. There's one
water pump in Ash, between sites 2
and 4; campers on other side of Ash
might want to use Birch water pump,
between sites 5 and 9.

site 11. Ash has six wheelchair-accessible sites (3–5 and 19–21). Next up is the Birch Loop (B) with 31 sites (sites 23 and 30 are reserved for camp hosts). There isn't much to distinguish the two loops except for the fact that Birch is home to an amphitheater. Again, this shouldn't be any concern at night, but daytime activities can make the sites nearest the amphitheater (28, specifi-cally) feel like epicenters of commotion.

Skip the Cedar Loop (C), as its 41 sites are for RVs, with full electrical hookups. The final loop is Dogwood (D). Even though Dogwood is the most crowded, with 60 sites (sites 22 and 32 are reserved for camp hosts), it's the farthest from the beach, lake, and campground entrance. It's also a decent distance from the RV loop at Cedar. But it's also nearest hunting areas, so if you're camping dur-ing hunting season, you may hear some gunshots, though they will seem far off. Sites 40–48, on the southern outside edge, offer the easiest access to the trails that access the AT. The same sites along the western edge (24–38) offer easiest access to the hiking trails in the hunt-ing area.

Greenbrier's campground is consis-tently well maintained and pretty. The

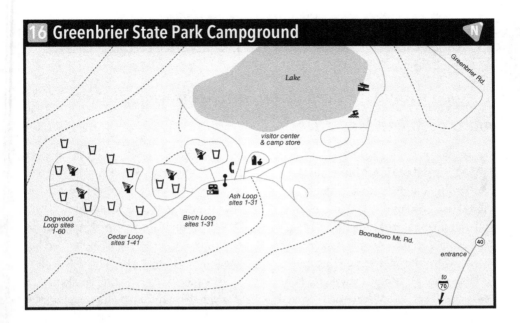

16 Greenbrier State Park Campground

Lake

visitor center & camp store

Dogwood Loop sites 1-60

Cedar Loop sites 1-41

Birch Loop sites 1-31

Ash Loop sites 1-31

Boonsboro Mt. Rd.

Greenbrier Rd.

entrance

40

to 70

only sites you may consider avoiding are those that sit closest to the entrance road: Ash: 1, 3, 5, 6, 8, 10, 26, 28, 30, 32; Birch: 1, 31; and Cedar: 1, 32, 33, 34, 36, 38, 40 (but you probably won't be in Cedar anyway). Dogwood is OK because the camp road ends there (or, more accurately, becomes the Dogwood Loop Road).

:: Getting There

From the east: Take I-70 West to Exit 42, MD 17. Bear right onto MD 17 North. Turn left onto US 40 West. Follow for 3 miles, and the park is on the left.

From the west: Take I-70 East to Exit 35, MD 66. Bear right onto MD 66. Turn left onto US 40 East and follow for 2 miles; the park is on the right.

GPS COORDINATES N39°32'10" W77°37'25"

17

Maple Tree Camp

The opportunity to sleep in a tree house is what attracts many people to Maple Tree.

The **Appalachian Mountain area** surrounding the 20-acre Maple Tree Camp has a bit of unpleasant history, both real and fictional. Here, on South Mountain, more than 6,000 soldiers were killed in the Civil War, effectively ending Robert E. Lee's 1862 Maryland incursion. Some 140 years later, a fictional witch lurked in these parts, which served as the home of *The Blair Witch Project*. The popular film brought a steady stream of visitors to nearby Burkittsville (a real town without a witch), convinced of the story's veracity. The thick woods surrounding the town aren't illusory, however, and provide a great setting for one of Maryland's most unusual camping opportunities.

The opportunity to sleep in a tree house (or tree cottage) is what attracts many people to Maple Tree. Each tree

house is enclosed, sits at least seven feet off the ground, and has a small deck. The largest among them, Falcon and Hawk, can accommodate up to 12 people. In addition to the tree houses, there's a log cabin, wooded tent sites, and field sites.

Maple Tree's location makes it a strategic base from which to explore the immediate area, which offers plenty of recreational activities. If you want history, Antietam National Battlefield—site of the single bloodiest battle in American history—and Harpers Ferry, West Virginia, are nearby but require a short drive to get there. Swimming and tubing on the Potomac are easy to do. Horseback riding can be arranged at the camp office. If the weather is crummy, go indoors to the fantastic Brunswick Railroad Museum in nearby Brunswick, or head underground at Crystal Grottoes Cavern just down the road from Antietam.

Of course, the area offers great hiking opportunities. Greenbrier, Washington Monument, and Gathland State Parks are nearby, as is Devil's Backbone County Park, home to hiking and fishing in Antietam Creek under the shadows of a beautiful stone bridge that survived the Civil War. Best of all, a portion of the

:: Ratings

BEAUTY: ★ ★ ★ ★
PRIVACY: ★ ★ ★ ★
SPACIOUSNESS: ★ ★ ★ ★
QUIET: ★ ★ ★
SECURITY: ★ ★ ★ ★ ★
CLEANLINESS: ★ ★ ★ ★

:: Key Information

ADDRESS: Maple Tree Camp
20716 Townsend Road
Rohrersville, MD 21779

CONTACT: 301-432-5585;
thetreehousecamp.com

OPERATED BY: Privately owned

OPEN: Year-round

SITES: 38+ total (10 tree cottages, 8 tree houses, 1 log cabin, 19 tent sites, plus field sites that can accommodate up to 60 campers)

EACH SITE: Wooded tent sites: fire circle, grill, picnic table; field sites: picnic table, fire circle

ASSIGNMENT: Reservations are recommended and honored for up to 4 days; 1-night deposit required; 2-night minimum on weekends

REGISTRATION: 301-432-5585 or **thetreehousecamp.com/reservations**

FACILITIES: Bathhouses, camp store, water, horseshoes, basketball hoop, pavilion

PARKING: At designated sites

FEE: Wooded tent sites $10/person, $30 minimum; field tent sites $8/person, $22 minimum; tree houses $43–$60/night for up to 4 people, $10 extra person; tree cottages $60–$74/night for up to 4 people, $10 extra person

RESTRICTIONS

▓ **Pets:** On leash

▓ **Quiet Hours:** 11 p.m.–7 a.m. (Seriously, a $250 "nuisance fee" can be incurred for egregious breaches.)

▓ **Visitors:** Fee above applies to all overnight visitors

▓ **Fires:** In fire rings

▓ **Alcohol:** Permitted

▓ **Stay Limit:** 2-night minimum weekends, except field sites; 3-night minimum Memorial and Labor Day weekends

▓ **Other:** All sites 50% off Wednesday

Appalachian Trail runs along the edge of the campground property. In fact, Maple Tree has become a popular stop for AT thru-hikers. Gathland State Park is just up the road from the turnoff to access Maple Tree; the unique Civil War Correspondent's Memorial is well worth the short hike there.

Maple Tree does not allow RVs or trailers, so it's generally quiet. The "wooded" tent sites are just that. Each, like the tree houses, affords a good amount of privacy and space. Tent sites range in size considerably, so when you make reservations, specify how many tents you have because different sites can accommodate anywhere from one to four tents. The website has a good campground map with this information as well. My favorite sites are those up the hill from the camp office, sitting by themselves in thick woods and a pristine setting: Lion, Leopard, Otter, Badger, and Wildebeest (grouped along a common entrance road); of these, Wildebeest, the last one reached, is the best, as it's completely isolated and has nothing but thick woods as its backyard. Beyond these are

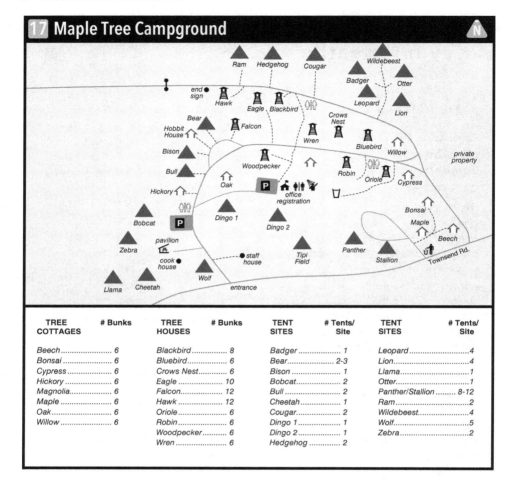

17 Maple Tree Campground

TREE COTTAGES	# Bunks	TREE HOUSES	# Bunks	TENT SITES	# Tents/Site	TENT SITES	# Tents/Site
Beech	6	Blackbird	8	Badger	1	Leopard	4
Bonsai	6	Bluebird	6	Bear	2-3	Lion	4
Cypress	6	Crows Nest	6	Bison	1	Llama	1
Hickory	6	Eagle	10	Bobcat	2	Otter	1
Magnolia	6	Falcon	12	Bull	2	Panther/Stallion	8-12
Maple	6	Hawk	12	Cheetah	1	Ram	2
Oak	6	Oriole	6	Cougar	2	Wildebeest	4
Willow	6	Robin	6	Dingo 1	1	Wolf	5
		Woodpecker	6	Dingo 2	1	Zebra	2
		Wren	6	Hedgehog	2		

three wonderful, isolated sites (my favorites): Cougar, Hedgehog, and Ram. If you don't get a wooded site, or if you prefer to look up at the stars, field sites are situated just in front of the camp office.

Maple Tree's campground is lovingly maintained by friendly and helpful owners, and it is truly a wonderful place, allowing for an easy getaway in an unspoiled setting. It's one of my favorites.

:: Getting There

Take I-70 to Frederick. Take Exit 52, US 340 West, and go 15 miles to MD 67 North toward Boonsboro. Go 5 miles and turn right on Gapland Road, and then turn left on Townsend Road.

GPS COORDINATES N39°24'37.4" W77°38'46.3"

18

New Germany State Park

New Germany is mountainous, unspoiled western Maryland—black bears, heavy snow, and all.

New Germany sits on the eastern side of the Continental Divide, but just barely. This makes it part of the Chesapeake watershed, a thought-provoking fact—if you're camping here, you'll feel a long way from Bay Country. This is mountainous, unspoiled western Maryland—black bears, heavy snow, and all. While it won't feel much like Chesapeake watershed, you probably won't be thinking of Germany either. The name of the area comes from the area's early settlers. Unfortunately, those folks completely cleared the forest, as was custom in the 1800s. By the middle of the next century, however, the land was turned over to the state, and the Civilian Conservation Corps began improvements. Now the forests have been replanted, and some sections soar with century-old trees. In

the park, the main attraction is 13-acre New Germany Lake, great for boating, fishing, and swimming. A result of damming, New Germany Lake contains bass, catfish, tiger muskie, and trout. These same fish species, as well as walleye, can be reeled in from Poplar Lick.

Autumn comes a bit early in these higher elevations, so snagging a campsite toward the end of the season is highly recommended. Aside from the thinning crowds, the fall foliage in the forest is simply spectacular. Gum, maple, and larch explode by October. Just remember, if you're coming from eastern Maryland, the nights here get surprisingly cool.

The campground is wooded and private. There are 47 campsites on three loops, plus one Alpine shelter. The first loop is the White Oak Loop, with sites 1–20 and 33–38. The Pines Loop is next, with sites 21–32 and 39. I really like site 39 because it sits by itself at the end of what appears to be a small gravel driveway. There's one potential catch, however—a short trail behind it leads to a parking lot. If people mistake this for a forest trail, you might get some company. A preferable site, if you can get it, is 40, easily the most

:: Ratings

BEAUTY: ★ ★ ★ ★
PRIVACY: ★ ★ ★
QUIET: ★ ★ ★
SPACIOUSNESS: ★ ★ ★
SECURITY: ★ ★ ★ ★ ★
CLEANLINESS: ★ ★ ★ ★ ★

:: Key Information

ADDRESS: New Germany State Park
349 Headquarters Lane
Grantsville, MD 21536

CONTACT: 301-895-5453;
dnr2.maryland.gov

OPERATED BY: Maryland Department
of Natural Resources

OPEN: Early April–late October

SITES: 48

EACH SITE: Picnic table, lantern post,
grill, camp pad

ASSIGNMENT: First come, first served
early September–end of the season;
reservations recommended otherwise

REGISTRATION: 888-432-CAMP
(2267) or **reservations.dnr.state.md.us**

FACILITIES: Bathhouses (no showers
early September–end of season), boat
rental, nature center, playground

PARKING: 2 vehicles/site

FEE: $18.49 plus service charge/night;
Memorial Day–Labor Day weekends
and holidays, $2/person day-use fee

RESTRICTIONS

▦ **Pets:** Permitted in the Hemlock
Loop, sites 50-58

▦ **Quiet Hours:** 11 p.m.–7 a.m.

▦ **Visitors:** Maximum 6 people/site

▦ **Fires:** In fire rings

▦ **Alcohol:** Permitted only inside
cabins and at shelters with valid
permit, as applicable

▦ **Stay Limit:** 2 weeks

private spot in the campground. It sits all by itself off the Pines Loop near Alpine Lodge. I also prefer the Pines Loop in general; as its name indicates, it's studded with pines, and the aroma is wonderful. Pines and White Oak share a bathhouse.

Sites 33 and 34 are close together, and 36 sits next to the bathhouse. Site 28 is nice, as it backs to thick woods. If stargazing is your thing, go for 29, which is open. Mostly every site is acceptable and promises quiet, as none are electric. For campers needing electricity, there are 10 camper cabins, all of them behind the nature center on a separate road from the camp loops. Cabin 3 is wheelchair accessible.

Hemlock Loop contains sites 51–57, and sits separately from White Oak and Pines. Because Hemlock is the smallest of the three loops, with the fewest sites, this perhaps makes it more preferable. The sites themselves aren't very distinguishable from those in the other loops, however.

Generally speaking, you'll be able to get a spot in New Germany if you're just popping in. Aside from four nonreservable sites (29–32), the overflow area allows for nine more camping sites. Trying to accommodate campers seems more the rule than the exception at New Germany. That said, a reservation is never a bad idea.

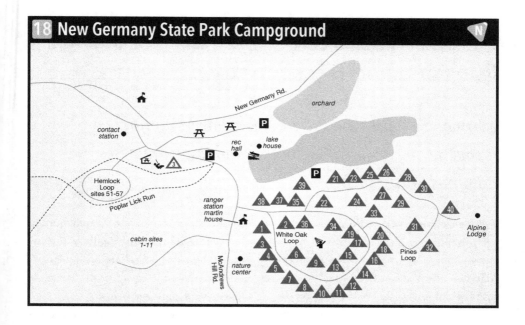

:: Getting There

Take Exit 22 off I-68 and follow Chestnut Ridge Road south to New Germany Road.

GPS COORDINATES N39°38'0" W79°7'17"

Potomac State Forest: Lostland Run Area and Backcountry Camping

Maryland's tallest mountain, Backbone Mountain, forms the northwest ridge of the land that comprises Potomac State Forest.

The **Potomac State Forest** is a special place, as it retains the vestiges of the wildness that used to make Western Maryland the first frontier for expansion-minded colonials. While the Allegheny Range of the Appalachian Mountains is puny by western standards, the mountains once proved a formidable obstacle to those heading west.

A friend of mine from Colorado scoffs at Maryland's "mountains," but I love my Appalachians. They are beautiful, rolling mountains, older by many centuries than the Rockies. Maryland's highest point, Backbone Mountain, forms the northwest ridge of the land that comprises Potomac State Forest. The summit of Backbone (3,360 feet) is farther to the

southeast, near the West Virginia border. But the ridge runs north, spilling its rainwater and snowmelt along several "runs" as they make their way to the Potomac River, some 1,000 feet below.

One of these waterways is the Lostland Run, which, along with the North Hill area, gives its name to Potomac State Forest's northern sections. In the Lostland Run Area, there's some great camping for those who want to get away from it all.

Following the directions, when you reach the Potomac Resource Center (Ranger Station), you will pass the trailhead for the Lostland Run Trail. This trail winds all the way to the incredible Potomac Overlook. It also winds close to each of the camping areas, paralleling the unpaved Lostland Run Road and traversing both the South Prong (of the Lostland Run) and North Prong suspension bridges. The trail is easily accessible from any of the camping sites in this area.

To get to the campsites, pass the headquarters of the Potomac Resource Center; take note of the picnic areas, bathrooms, and water nearby. Farther

:: Ratings

BEAUTY: ★ ★ ★ ★ ★
PRIVACY: ★ ★ ★ ★ ★
SPACIOUSNESS: ★ ★ ★ ★ ★
QUIET: ★ ★ ★ ★ ★
SECURITY: ★ ★ ★
CLEANLINESS: ★ ★ ★ ★ ★

:: Key Information

ADDRESS: Potomac State Forest
1431 Potomac Camp Road
Oakland, MD 21550

CONTACT: 301-334-2038;
dnr2.maryland.gov

OPERATED BY: Maryland Department
of Natural Resources

OPEN: Year-round, but roads are not
maintained in winter

SITES: 6+ (6 in Lostland Run Area, plus
one lean-to and one group site, which
holds a maximum of 20 campers, plus
unlimited in forest backcountry)

EACH SITE: Lantern hook, grill, picnic
table (Lostland Run Area)

ASSIGNMENT: First come, first served;
group sites must be reserved

REGISTRATION: Self-registration
stations at the entrance to each area;
for group sites, call 301-334-2038.

FACILITIES: Group sites have sanita-
tion facilities but no potable water.

PARKING: Vehicles must be parked on
gravel portion of site, off road in forest

FEE: $10/night, $15 lean-to shelter,
$20 group

RESTRICTIONS

▮ **Pets:** Permitted

▮ **Quiet Hours:** 11 p.m.–7 a.m.

▮ **Visitors:** Maximum 8 people or 2
units (20 people for group sites)

▮ **Fires:** In fire rings

▮ **Alcohol:** Permitted only inside
cabins and at shelters with valid
permit, as applicable

▮ **Stay Limit:** 2 weeks

▮ **Other:** Checkout 3 p.m. for roadside
sites. This is bear country—take proper
precautions. For tips on how to camp
among bears, visit **dnr.state.md.us
/wildlife/HuntTrap/blackbear/bbliving
with.asp.** Camping prohibited within
200 feet of any trail or stream.

along Potomac Camp Road, you'll see the unpaved Lostland Run Road to the right. The self-registration station is just up ahead. The first site along the road is 30. Like all the established sites in the state forest, it's spacious, private, and located in a beautiful natural setting—you can't go wrong with any of the sites along the road. Which you choose should depend mostly on vacancy and how much bumpy driving you're willing to endure to make your way along Lostland Run Road. The farther you go, the closer you get to the Potomac River, if that appeals.

As part of a group site, there is another picnic area (marked T-35) and toilet just beyond site 30; site 31 is just ahead as well. Then it's a good distance to the next site, almost a full mile. It's a jarring ride down the unpaved road, and even though getting closer to the river might be desirable, taking the trail there on foot is the much more pleasurable way to arrive. However, it might be worth the car trip down this road because just after site 32 is a lean-to shelter site; like the same in the other sections of the Potomac State Forest (see pages 78–80), these sites are well worth

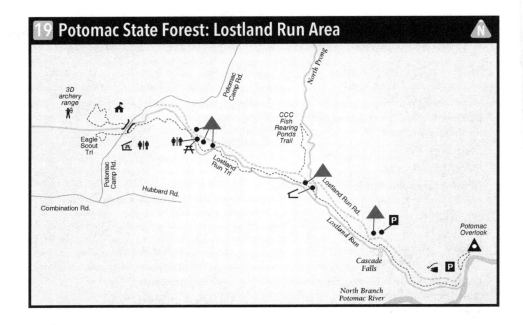

19 Potomac State Forest: Lostland Run Area

3D archery range

Eagle Scout Trl

Potomac Camp Rd.

Potomac Camp Rd.

CCC Fish Rearing Ponds Trail

North Prong

Lostland Run Trl

Hubbard Rd.

Combination Rd.

Lostland Run Rd.

Lostland Run

Cascade Falls

Potomac Overlook

North Branch Potomac River

the extra $5. If you're suddenly hit with a deluge during the night, it's nice to have the luxury of settling into the shelter.

If you're still making your way down Lostland Run Road and you've passed the shelter, you only have one more choice for a campsite, site 34. I wouldn't expect all the sites to be taken, as this area is pretty remote. However, if you find this is the case—or you want an even more backcountry experience—you are allowed to camp in any primitive setting in the state forest so long as you don't pitch your tent within 200 feet of a trail or stream. Backcountry permits can be obtained through the self-registration stations at Lostland Run or Laurel Run/Wallman (see pages 78–80).

If you do desire backcountry camping, you can either venture off the main

arteries described above or into the North Hill area, a wild and rugged section of the state forest north of Lostland Run. To reach it, stay on Potomac Camp Road, passing the turnoff for the Lostland Run area, and follow Potomac Camp to a right on North Hill Road. Be on the lookout about 0.2 mile later for the North Hill Trail, a small tertiary road. Once here, you'll find places to leave the car (take care not to block the passage) and set off into deep, untamed, unmarked forest.

There are two more forest areas ripe for backcountry camping. Following the directions above for North Hill, you can bypass North Hill Road and instead head left onto Upperman Road. When Upperman intersects with Eagle Rock Road, take a left; this quadrant of forest, to the south and east, is all prime camping area. Last, the Wallman Area (see pages 78–80) runs pretty far south of the main campsites. Loop Road, Bradshaw Hollow Road, and Trestle Road (nearest the Potomac) can all be accessed by heading south from Wallman Road, and you can camp in the forest anywhere off these roads.

:: Getting There

From Oakland, take MD 135 east to MD 560 and turn right. Go 3 miles to a left on Bethlehem Road. (Stay on Bethlehem at the intersection to Eagle Rock Road.) Go left on Combination Road and left on Potomac Camp Road. Pass the Potomac Resource Center, and the self-registration station is on Lostland Run Road.

GPS COORDINATES N39°22'55.0" W79°16'40.8"

20

Potomac State Forest:
Laurel Run and Wallman Areas

The cliffs that overlook the Potomac are impressive and offer endless opportunities for sightseeing.

The Potomac State Forest encompasses more than 11,000 acres of pristine wilderness bordering the North Branch of the Potomac River. The forest also includes portions of Backbone Mountain, Maryland's highest point. While the summit of Backbone sits outside of the state forest, sections within the forest exceed 3,000 feet. Both the Wallman and Laurel Run areas maintain elevation levels of 2,000–2,700 feet.

Like much of Maryland's western forests, the entire area was once denuded but has been allowed to grow back naturally and now serves as a protected area for an abundance of wildlife, including a thriving population of black bears. There are well-marked trails all throughout this rugged mountain wilderness; the state forest provides for some ideal backcountry camping. The cliffs that overlook the Potomac are impressive and offer endless opportunities for sightseeing.

Follow the directions; when Audley Riley Road becomes unpaved, you'll see the self-registration station. The road splits here; left is Laurel Run Road, right is Wallman Road, both unpaved.

Laurel Run Road heads east and ends at a fishing spot on the North Branch of the Potomac River. Because of the condition of the road, it makes for a long drive. Be prepared for the jarring the roads will inflict on your car. You might be tempted to stop at the first campsite you come to so as to avoid more jarring. This wouldn't be such a terrible thing. The first site, 20, is a good indicator of the campsites all along Laurel Run Road—spacious, roomy, and in a beautiful setting. Your only reasons for venturing beyond this site are if it's already taken or if you wish to be nearer the river. If you want to push on, the next site, 21, is the only one of the 10 sites along Laurel Run Road that has a

:: Ratings

BEAUTY: ★ ★ ★ ★ ★
PRIVACY: ★ ★ ★ ★ ★
SPACIOUSNESS: ★ ★ ★ ★ ★
QUIET: ★ ★ ★ ★ ★
SECURITY: ★ ★ ★
CLEANLINESS: ★ ★ ★ ★ ★

:: Key Information

ADDRESS: Potomac State Forest
1431 Potomac Camp Road
Oakland, MD 21550

CONTACT: 301-334-2038;
dnr2.maryland.gov

OPERATED BY: Maryland Department
of Natural Resources

OPEN: Year-round, but roads are not
maintained in winter

SITES: 16 (10 at Laurel Run,
6 at Wallman)

EACH SITE: Lantern hook, grill,
picnic table

ASSIGNMENT: First come, first served;
group sites must be reserved

REGISTRATION: Self-registration
stations at the entrance to each area;
for group sites, call 301-334-2038.

FACILITIES: Group sites have sanita-
tion facilities but no potable water.

PARKING: Vehicles must be parked on
gravel portion of site.

FEE: $10/night, $15 lean-to shelter,
$20 group

RESTRICTIONS

▨ **Pets:** Permitted

▨ **Quiet Hours:** 11 p.m.–7 a.m.

▨ **Visitors:** Maximum 8 people or 2
units (20 people for group sites)

▨ **Fires:** In fire rings

▨ **Alcohol:** Permitted only inside
cabins and at shelters with valid
permit, as applicable

▨ **Stay Limit:** 2 weeks

▨ **Other:** Checkout 3 p.m. This is bear
country–take proper precautions. For
tips on how to camp among bears,
visit **dnr.state.md.us/wildlife/Hunt
Trap/blackbear/bblivingwith.asp.**

lean-to shelter. Built in 2000 and called the Laurel Run Lodge (a bit of a misnomer), it's solidly constructed. If there's a chance of horrendous weather, why not give yourself the security of having the shelter to duck into if need be? Even if you never use the shelter, the site itself is extraordinary. Laurel Run (a beautiful rocky river) flows just behind the site, along with a narrow hiking trail.

After that, the sites are more or less the same—roomy, private, and in a spectacular natural setting; you really can't go wrong with any one of them. Be aware that while the first three campsites come

relatively quickly one after the other (assuming you're traveling by car), the next one (site 22) is half a mile away. It's followed quickly by sites 23, 24, and 25, which also sit near one another, about a tenth of a mile farther east on Laurel Run Road. There are two more sites along the road, and the last one (site 27) sits about half a mile from the river.

Back at the self-registration station, if you head right along Wallman Road, the first thing you come to is a large campsite (40). It's followed by two picnic areas, a group site, and a bathroom off Loop Road; Loop Road eventually

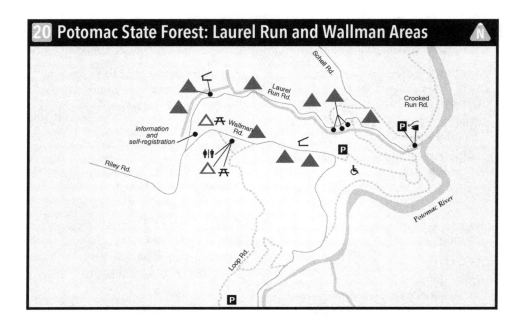

20 Potomac State Forest: Laurel Run and Wallman Areas

heads deep into the wilds of the forested Wallman Area. You'll notice that the group sites are not that much bigger than the single sites. Beyond the group sites, there are four more campsites, all in relatively quick succession. The third one is a shelter site like the one in the Laurel Run section described above; if it's available, grab it.

Of the two areas, I prefer Laurel Run over Wallman, as it feels a bit more wooded to me. If you want river access, Laurel Run is the better option as well.

Where Wallman Road makes a sharp right after the final campsite, there's a parking area straight ahead and a Disabled Hunter Access Road that leads to Trestle Road (all unpaved). You'd have to take a left on Trestle and make your way to Laurel Run Road to get down to the river.

My preference for Laurel Run is a subjective one—the truth is that camping in the Potomac State Forest is fantastic wherever you wind up. If you're looking for an accessible backcountry camping experience, you're sure to enjoy it.

:: Getting There

From Oakland, take MD 135 east to MD 560 and turn right. Go 3.5 miles to a left on White Church-Steyer Road. Go left on Audley Riley Road to the self-registration station.

GPS COORDINATES   N39°20'16.6" W79°18'32.5"

21

Rocky Gap State Park

A hemlock stand within the gorge is a sight to behold.

Rocky Gap State Park can, admittedly, turn off some rugged individualists. After all, it's not just a state park, but rather an entire complex, complete with resort, hotel, casino, golf course, and restaurants. Though the land was settled in 1730, the modern park was established in 1974 and was the brainchild of an Allegany County congressman. Its intent was to draw tourists and create jobs, but that plan hasn't always worked out. For years, the resort struggled to make money.

Many first-time campers at Rocky Gap seeking to get away from it all are horrified when they enter the park and see the sprawling complex before them. But take heart: the park itself contains more than 3,000 acres, including 243-acre Lake Habeeb, and planners had the good sense to at least build the resort and golf course on the side of the lake

:: Ratings

BEAUTY: ★ ★ ★ ★
PRIVACY: ★ ★ ★
SPACIOUSNESS: ★ ★ ★
QUIET: ★ ★
SECURITY: ★ ★ ★ ★
CLEANLINESS: ★ ★ ★ ★ ★

opposite the campgrounds. So, although you have to drive through the resort area to get to your campsite, once there you will enjoy relative solitude (as much as a campground with 278 sites can offer).

Even better, hiking away from the lake will leave all the bustle behind and you'll likely see few people as you make your way around Evitts Mountain, named for the settler who built his cabin here in the 1730s. Two 500-acre tracts have been designated as state wildlands and are truly beautiful, full of foxes, black bears, white-tailed deer—and the more elusive bobcats as well. A hemlock stand within the gorge is also a site to behold.

Rocky Gap has nine camp loops, each corresponding to its first letter—A for Ash, B for Birch, C for Chestnut, etc. The others are Dogwood, Elm, Fir, Gum, Hickory, and Ironwood. Ash, with its 30 sites, is entirely electric. Birch, Chestnut, and Dogwood all intersect and are close to one another. While individual sites are often separated by 50 or more feet of nice tree buffers, don't expect to feel alone in any of these loops unless you're here midweek or in the off-season. If you do stay in one of these three loops (bathhouses are within Dogwood and Chestnut), I'd

:: Key Information

ADDRESS: Rocky Gap State Park
17600 Campers Hill Road
Flintstone, MD 21530

CONTACT: 301-722-1480;
dnr2.maryland.gov

OPERATED BY: Maryland Department
of Natural Resources

OPEN: Year-round, with limited services from Columbus Day to the first
Friday in May

SITES: 278

EACH SITE: Picnic table, fire ring

ASSIGNMENT: reservations recommended between May and Columbus
Day

REGISTRATION: 888-432-CAMP
(2267) or **reservations.dnr.state.md.us**

FACILITIES: Dump station, bathhouses,
boat ramp and rentals, laundry, camp
store, nature center, game room,
swimming beach, pay phones

PARKING: On gravel driveway

FEE: $21.49 plus service charge/night,
$27.49 plus service charge/night elec-
tric; additional day-use service charge
during high season $4–$6

RESTRICTIONS

▨ **Pets:** Allowed in Ash, Birch, Chestnut, Dogwood, and Elm Loops (sites
1–143) and common areas

▨ **Quiet Hours:** 11 p.m.–7 a.m.

▨ **Visitors:** Check-in at registration
desk

▨ **Fires:** In fire rings

▨ **Alcohol:** Permitted only inside
cabins and at shelters with valid
permit, as applicable

▨ **Stay Limit:** Maximum 10 consecutive days

▨ **Other:** Checkout 3 p.m.

recommend the western edge of Dogwood, specifically sites 91 and 92 or those
close by. These sites are bounded by
woods (Chestnut bounds the other side
of the loop) and sit astride the wonderful
Evitts Mountain Homesite Trail, accessed
by using the lovely Rocky Trail. If you
don't feel alone, you can take a few steps
and achieve solitude.

Elm Loop (sites 111–143) offers easy
access to the camp store and sits near
the lake, so if water sports are more your
thing, this might be a good option. It's
also closest to the Lakeside Loop Trail, a

challenging and rewarding path around
the shoreline. Sites 120–127 are closest to
the lake. Gum (sites 175–204) and Hickory
(sites 205–237) are next; Hickory would
be my suggestion, as this loop is tent-only
(while only Ash is electric, all other loops
apart from Hickory accommodate RVs).
The southern sites in Hickory (232–237)
are near the group camping area. Conse-
quently, these can be noisier than others.
Sites 220–228 on the northwest corner of
Hickory also provide easy access to the
southern portion of the Evitts Mountain
Homesite Trail.

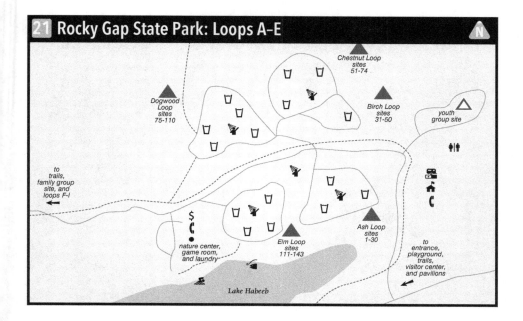

21 Rocky Gap State Park: Loops A–E

Chestnut Loop
sites
51–74

Dogwood
Loop
sites
75–110

Birch Loop
sites
31–50

youth
group site

to
trails,
family group
site, and
loops F–I

nature center,
game room,
and laundry

Elm Loop
sites
111–143

Ash Loop
sites
1–30

to
entrance,
playground,
trails,
visitor center,
and pavilions

Lake Habeeb

Lastly, Fir (sites 144–174) and Ironwood (239–278) are often the most popular because of their proximity to Lake Habeeb. Sites 156–166 in Fir and 255–265 in Ironwood are closest to the lake, with 256–260 nearest the dock. Ironwood also offers easy access to the Lakeside Loop Trail, which is the most popular in the park. Again, my recommendation is to head farther away from the lake and toward the less used, more pleasant loops, concentrating your search on Hickory. You can always check out the lake after you're down from the mountain.

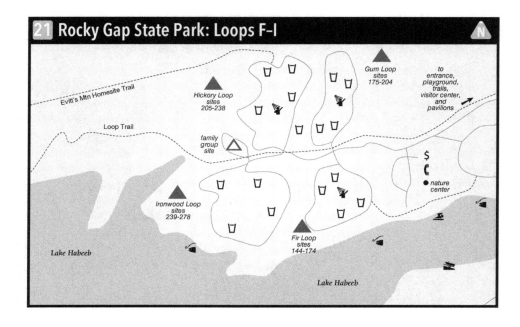

:: Getting There

Take I-68 to Exit 50/Rocky Gap State Park; you'll see it right away. To reach the campground, turn right onto Pleasant Valley Road and travel 1.5 miles.

GPS COORDINATES   N39°41'58" W78°40'24"

22

Savage River State Forest:
Whitewater, Big Run, and Savage River Road Campsites

What makes the campsites in the state forest unique is that most guarantee almost total privacy.

Things can get a bit confusing in these parts, with so many nearby and often congruous parks—including Big Run (pages 12–14) and New Germany (pages 71–73)—and recreation areas, all contained within the 54,000-acre Savage River Forest. What makes the campsites in the state forest unique is that most guarantee almost total privacy. The Savage River sites spread like tentacles near and around Big Run and New Germany state parks and the Savage River Reservoir. Savage River Forest is Maryland's largest protected site, and it includes some 12,000 acres of wildlands, which earn special protections. There are some 100 miles of

trails throughout the forest, allowing you to pick a length and configuration and go.

Fishing and boating are also popular in the forest. Interestingly, its two main rivers, Savage and Casselman, end up in very different places: Savage heads to the Potomac and eventually ends up in the Atlantic, while Casselman sits on the western side of the continental divide, heads to the Youghiogheny, and eventually empties its waters in the Mississippi. Many regard these rivers and native trout streams as the best trout fisheries in the state. The reservoir itself is a major draw and sees many boaters and anglers. But the forest's location in a relatively remote portion of the state ensures that it never feels overrun.

I've split the forest camping into two entries in this book, in large part because it can take surprisingly long to drive around this vast and largely untouched area; much of Savage River Road, for instance, offers an absolutely beautiful ride, one which will undoubtedly compel you to stop the car and head down to

:: Ratings

BEAUTY: ★ ★ ★ ★ ★
PRIVACY: ★ ★ ★ ★
SPACIOUSNESS: ★ ★ ★ ★
QUIET: ★ ★ ★ ★
SECURITY: ★ ★ ★ ★
CLEANLINESS: ★ ★ ★ ★ ★

:: Key Information

ADDRESS: Savage River State Forest 127 Headquarters Lane Grantsville, MD 21536

CONTACT: 301-895-5759; **dnr2.maryland.gov**

OPERATED BY: Maryland Department of Natural Resources

OPEN: Year-round

SITES: 36, plus backcountry camping

EACH SITE: Picnic table, fire ring, tent pad

ASSIGNMENT: First come, first served

REGISTRATION: Self-register within first hour of arrival by filling out a form, paying, and placing both in one of the self-registration standpipes. Locations are on Savage River Road, southeast of the reservoir at the Whitewater Campsites (114–122); on Savage River Road between Big Run State Park and site 113; and on Big Run Road near New Germany Road, just after site 144. Self-register for backcountry camping at any of the six self-registration sites (see other Savage River SF entry in this book for the location of the other three self-registration sites). Enclose a trip itinerary and the names of the people in your party if backcountry camping.

FACILITIES: Boat launches

PARKING: Maximum 2 vehicles/site; must be parked in entrance drive or camping pad

FEE: $15/night numbered sites; $10/night backcountry

RESTRICTIONS

▧ **Pets:** Permitted on a leash

▧ **Quiet Hours:** 11 p.m.–7 a.m.

▧ **Visitors:** Maximum 6 people and 2 tents/site

▧ **Fires:** Allowed in fire rings but not within the 12,000 acres of the Wildlands areas if backcountry camping; consult a park map available at headquarters.

▧ **Alcohol:** Permitted only inside cabins and at shelters with valid permit, as applicable

▧ **Stay Limit:** Each numbered site must be reserved daily.

▧ **Other:** This is bear country—take proper precautions. For tips on how to camp among bears, visit **dnr.state .md.us/wildlife/HuntTrap/blackbear /bblivingwith.asp.**

the water. This entry covers the camping areas immediately northeast, northwest, and southeast of the reservoir, numbered 106–144. These are your best bets if proximity to the reservoir is what you desire.

Sites 114–122, the Whitewater Campsites, are southeast of the reservoir, along Savage River Road, and not far from the Savage River Dam, on the southeasternmost edge of the reservoir. These sites

are popular, as they sit near the reservoir and offer easy access to the boat launch on its southern end. Also, they're easy to get to, as Savage River Road is paved and the sites sit right off the road. However, they don't offer much privacy because they're near one another and aren't heavily wooded. But a bonus is that these sites sit near the Savage River, which is crossable here because of its proximity to the

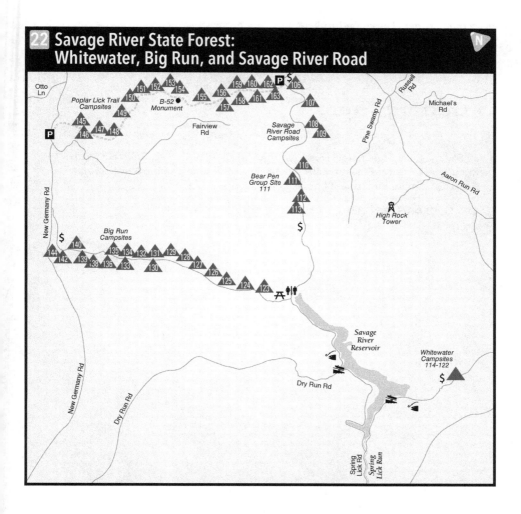

22 Savage River State Forest: Whitewater, Big Run, and Savage River Road

dam. That's a good thing because the Big Savage hiking trail, 17 miles in length, is easily accessible in the woods just to the north of the campsites and the river.

To the northwest of the reservoir sits Big Run Road, where you'll find sites 123–144, in that order, heading northwest toward New Germany Road. There isn't too much to distinguish these sites; every one is essentially the same size and

uniform in their distance from Big Run Road and its namesake, Big Run. Basically, if one of these sites looks good to you, just take the first one that's vacant (just don't forget to register for it).

If instead of moving northwest along Big Run, you went northeast, you'd first pass Big Run State Park (see pages 12–14), and then, heading along Savage River Drive, you'd pass sites 113–106, in descending order. These tend to be a little more spaced out from one another in comparison to those along Big Run road to the west but are otherwise similar. Note also that one group site, 111, is among this cluster.

:: Getting There

To Savage River State Forest Headquarters: Take I-68 to Exit 22, Chestnut Ridge Road/US 219 toward Meyersdale. Go 2.6 miles and turn left onto New Germany Road. Go 2 miles and turn right onto Headquarters Lane.

GPS COORDINATES **Headquarters:** N39°37'49.8" W79°07'51.7"

23

Savage River State Forest:
Elk Lick, Poplar Lick, and Blue Lick Campsites

Enjoy easy access to the pristine forest and a remote experience here.

As explained in the previous entry, I've split the Savage River State Forest camping into two for this book: This entry takes in the areas to the far north of the Savage River Reservoir, but closer to the forest headquarters and I-68, providing easier access in and out. In this more mountainous, wooded location, you won't be near the reservoir itself, but you will have easy access to the pristine forest. The campsites located here provide a year-round and inexpensive alternative to New Germany State Park. Plus, compared to New Germany, the Savage River sites give a more backcountry, remote feel to your camping experience. While amenities like those at New

Germany are nice, for me the seclusion of the Savage River State Forest campsites beats a maintained campground any day.

Campsites in this section are spread along Westernport Road in the Elk Lick Area, along the Poplar Lick Off-Road Vehicle (ORV) Trail heading south toward Savage River Road and the reservoir, and the small Blue Lick section off Lower New Germany Road near Blue Lick Run. (Incidentally, the state forest headquarters and New Germany State Park are only a few miles to the west.)

First, Poplar Lick: If you were heading south along New Germany Road from New Germany State Park and the state forest headquarters, you'd soon see a little dirt road just after the New Germany store. A sign there indicates Poplar Lick ORV Trail. The first site you'll come to, on the left, is site 145. Another 18 sites (146–163) follow the trail until it reaches Savage River Road. These are nice sites, much like the state forest campsites at Garrett and Potomac—generally a cleared space in the forest just off the road or trail and studded with trees. They are large, very

:: Ratings

BEAUTY: ★ ★ ★ ★ ★
PRIVACY: ★ ★ ★ ★
SPACIOUSNESS: ★ ★ ★
QUIET: ★ ★ ★ ★ ★
SECURITY: ★ ★ ★ ★
CLEANLINESS: ★ ★ ★ ★ ★

:: Key Information

ADDRESS: Savage River State Forest 127 Headquarters Lane Grantsville, MD 21536

CONTACT: 301-895-5759; **dnr2.maryland.gov**

OPERATED BY: Maryland Department of Natural Resources

OPEN: Year-round

SITES: 30, plus backcountry camping

EACH SITE: Picnic table, fire ring, tent pad

ASSIGNMENT: First come, first served

REGISTRATION: Self-register within first hour of arrival by filling out a form, paying, and placing both in one of the self-registration standpipes. Locations are at Savage River State Headquarters at New Germany Road near McAndrews Hill Road; Elk Lick Run on Westernport Road at the Elk Lick Campsites (standpipe is nearest site 100); and on Savage River Road near site 106 at the entrance to the Poplar Lick campsites. Self-register for backcountry camping at any of the six self-registration sites (see other Savage River SF entry in this book for the location of the other three self-registration sites). Enclose a trip itinerary and the names of the people in your party if backcountry camping.

FACILITIES: Boat launches

PARKING: Maximum 2 vehicles/site; vehicles must be parked in entrance drive or camping pad

FEE: $15/night numbered sites; $10/night backcountry

RESTRICTIONS

▓ **Pets:** Permitted on a leash

▓ **Quiet Hours:** 11 p.m.–7 a.m.

▓ **Visitors:** Maximum 6 people and 2 tents/site

▓ **Fires:** Allowed in fire rings but not within the 12,000 acres of the Wildlands areas if backcountry camping

▓ **Alcohol:** Permitted only inside cabins and at shelters with valid permit, as applicable

▓ **Stay Limit:** Each numbered site must be reserved daily.

▓ **Other:** This is bear country–take proper precautions. For tips on how to camp among bears, visit **dnr.state .md.us/wildlife/HuntTrap/blackbear /bblivingwith.asp.**

private, and well wooded. There is one reason for hesitation when it comes to these sites, however—this is an ORV trail, and off-road vehicles can mean noise. Although ORVs (trucks and vehicles with four- or all-wheel drive) are less noisy and smelly than all-terrain vehicles, any passing vehicle's capacity for spoiling your solitude and peacefulness depends entirely on the driver's speed and general courtesy.

Parking areas can be found near Savage River Road at site 163 and near New Germany Road, closest to site 145. The 6-mile Poplar Lick Trail is simply beautiful. It is what remains of a 1934 Civilian Conservation Corps road, and it boasts a riot of wildflowers in the summer months.

Closer to New Germany State Park are the six sites along Westernport Road, which you can reach by following the

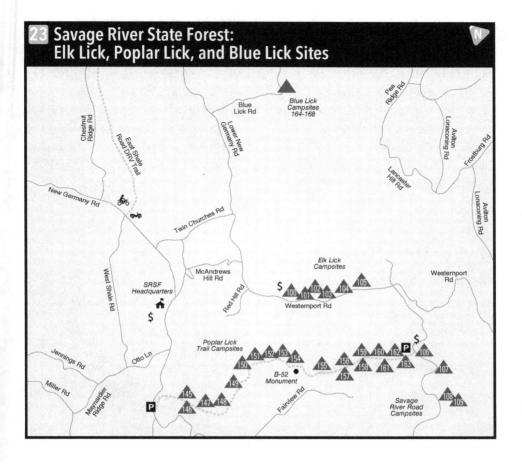

23 Savage River State Forest: Elk Lick, Poplar Lick, and Blue Lick Sites

directions to New Germany State Park and then either going through the park on McAndrews Hill Road or just north of the park on Twin Churches Road and then heading right (south) on Westernport. The campsites (100–105) sit along Westernport just before you reach Savage River Road. These sites are much easier to get to than those along the Poplar Lick Trail, so if you have a smallish vehicle, these might be your better bets. Further, because of their proximity to Savage River Road (what constitutes a "major" road in

these parts), you can easily access the reservoir by heading south.

For Blue Lick, the farthest entries for this camping area, take Westernport Road north from McAndrews or Twin Churches and follow it to Lower New Germany Road north to a right on Blue Lick Road for sites 164–168.

There are two more camping areas within the forest, both of which are, in the words of a helpful ranger, seldom used because they lack access to water. They are primitive and remote and don't show up on campground maps. They are used primarily by deer hunters but are accessible and fall under the same rules and procedures as the rest of the sites within the forest. These sites are found in two different locations. The first location can be accessed off I-68, Exit 19 (US 219 South). Go about 2 miles to a left on Rabbit Hollow Road, where the sites are located. This area is called the Margraff Trails area, used mostly by hunters from the nearby town of Accident. The other location is at Keysers Ridge, on Negro Mountain (elevation more than 3,000 feet and named in the 18th century to honor an African American fighter in the French and Indian War). It can also be reached by taking Exit 14, but going north instead to US 40 West. Look for Keysers Ridge Road as a dirt track north (right) of US 40.

:: Getting There

To Savage River Road southeast of the reservoir: Take I-68 to Exit 34, MD 36 (New Georges Creek Road) south toward Luke. Go 15 miles west on MD 135, then another 2 miles, and head right (northwest) onto Savage River Road. To Savage River State Forest Headquarters: See previous entry.

GPS COORDINATES   Headquarters: N39°37'49.8" W79°07'51.7"

24

South Mountain State Park:
Appalachian Trail Shelters

The great ideal of the AT is its accessibility to everyone willing to give it a go.

South Mountain State Park isn't your traditional park in that there is no actual headquarters or entrance facility, nor even clear boundary lines. Instead, this park encompasses the 40 miles and 13,000 acres of forest along the ridge of South Mountain that contain Maryland's portion of the Appalachian Trail. (The Appalachian Trail itself is blazed in white; blue blazes indicate trails to the shelters where you can pitch your tent.) Prominent signage makes finding the shelters easy. Aside from the three backpackers-only campgrounds (see pages 97–99), people are prohibited from camping along the trail—except in the designated shelters listed here—or near

them. It should go without saying that you must be extremely careful to leave no trace when camping at these areas.

Mindfulness is in order when planning a camping trip in South Mountain along the AT. After all, South Mountain State Park doesn't advertise itself as a camping destination; the understanding is that the six primitive shelters and camping areas within the park are primarily for AT thru-hikers. True, perhaps one who has hiked from Maine or Georgia and eventually arrives in Maryland should have dibs on the campsites, but there's nothing wrong with locals who are hiking just the Maryland section—no small undertaking in itself—using the camping sites as well.

There are six primitive shelters along the Maryland portion of the AT. From north to south, they are: Raven Rock (0.2 mile from Pen Mar, near the Pennsylvania border), Ensign Cowall, Pine Knob, Rocky Run, Crampton Gap, and Ed Garvey, which is 3.5 miles north of the C&O Canal and the Potomac River. All six shelters look fairly similar: generally smallish,

:: Ratings

BEAUTY: ★ ★ ★ ★ ★
PRIVACY: ★ ★ ★
SPACIOUSNESS: ★ ★ ★
QUIET: ★ ★ ★
SECURITY: ★ ★ ★
CLEANLINESS: ★ ★ ★ ★

:: Key Information

ADDRESS: South Mountain State Park
c/o South Mountain Recreation Area
21843 National Pike
Boonsboro, MD 21713

CONTACT: South Mountain State Park:
301-791-4767, **dnr2.maryland.gov**;
Appalachian National Scenic Trail
NPS Park Office: 304-535-6278,
nps.gov/appa

OPERATED BY: South Mountain State
Park is operated by the Maryland
Department of Natural Resources; the
Appalachian Trail is operated by the
National Park Service and a consor-
tium of local hiking and conservation
organizations.

OPEN: Year-round

SITES: Shelters hold 6–12 people; each
site allows for additional tent sites

EACH SITE: Picnic table, fire ring, privy

ASSIGNMENT: First come, first served

REGISTRATION: None

FACILITIES: Toilet (some have spring
water)

PARKING: None

FEE: Free

RESTRICTIONS

■ **Pets:** Permitted on a leash

■ **Quiet Hours:** Officially none

■ **Visitors:** The Appalachian Trail Conservancy suggests hiking and camping in groups no larger than 10
people.

■ **Fires:** In fire rings

■ **Alcohol:** Not permitted

■ **Stay Limit:** Practice and hikers'
etiquette dictate short stays of 1–2
days during warmer months when
demand is highest.

■ **Other:** Allow thru-hikers first use of
shelters

hewn-log structures sitting amid comparatively level ground (the areas around
the shelters are invariably hilly).

Because the overnight parking area
just off US 40 and adjacent to I-70 is easy
to get to and is the Maryland AT's almost
midpoint, I'll operate under the assump-
tion that trips to the shelters begin from
there. The closest shelter site to this area
is Pine Knob, which sits just 0.5 mile to
the north. To reach the shelter, go west
0.1 mile from the AT on the blue-blazed
trail (don't cross I-70 on the bridge, but

rather head right just down from the
parking area).

In the first edition of this book, I
wrote: "Those wishing to pitch a tent at
Pine Knob might find it a bit disappoint-
ing. It's often served as a partying spot,
and it shows, with discarded beer cans and
the like." I'm happy to report that on subsequent trips to Pine Knob, I have found
it clean and looking nice. There's a lot of
cleared space, so making do isn't so tough.
The biggest downfall of this shelter is that
you can hear I-70 in the distance. But its

location provides some major pluses: both Greenbrier State Park (see pages 65–67) and George Washington State Park are nearby. The biggest nearby attraction is the short hike to Annapolis Rock, a beautiful perch that allows great vistas. Signage to Annapolis Rock is easy to spot and follow.

Continuing north: Ensign Cowall is 8.2 miles from Pine Knob. Ensign Cowall is an attractive structure, with a pitched wood roof and some handsome triangular windows. It has level ground nearby to pitch a tent.

The last shelter in this direction is at Raven Rock, which, in 2010, replaced the oft-bemoaned Devils Racecourse Shelter. The lovely and still relatively new Raven Rock is 5 miles north of Ensign Cowall, a few hundred yards from the turnoff for Devils Racecourse (the site, not the shelter, now long gone), a boulder field situated between rows of mature trees. If the haul from the US 40/I-70 parking area is too far, you can reach this portion of the trail from MD 491 in Cascade and find overnight parking 5 miles north of the shelter at the Pen Mar County Park. One word of caution to those who remember the Devils Racecourse shelter: the spring that was there is now gone, as well, and there is no new water source at Raven Rock.

If you're heading south from the US 40/I-70 parking area, the first shelter along the route is Rocky Run, which is 6.9 miles south. (To reach the shelter, go west for 0.2 mile on the blue-blazed trail.) There are actually two shelters at Rocky Run, one

only a few years old (and wonderful) and the older one that was extensively repaired in 2008. There is also a new privy. This is a wonderful spot. Indeed, Rocky Run is one of my favorites: the setting is pristine, there's lots of space to camp (for level ground, head up the hill from the shelter to the fire pit), and a pipe sends clear, delicious spring water rushing out of the rocky hill. The only drawback here is that if you're tenting just outside of the shelter, the ground is pretty rocky.

Crampton Gap is next, 5 miles from Rocky Run. AT thru-hikers often find Crampton Gap a pleasure—it's a bit snug, but it has an outhouse and a nice deck. The downside is the rocky terrain—clearing a space for your tent takes a bit of maneuvering. Another access option for Crampton Gap is the overnight parking area at the Civil War Correspondents' Memorial on Gapland Road (MD 572), 1 mile west of Burkittsville.

Last is Ed Garvey, 4.1 miles from Crampton Gap. Ed Garvey is beautifully constructed. On approach, it looks more like a ski lodge than a primitive camping shelter. Picnic tables and massive crisscrossed logs make it an attractive place. Additionally, there's plenty of space for a tent, both right next to the shelter and on the little trails adjacent to it. Ed Garvey allows easy access to Weverton Cliffs, which gives great views over the Potomac River and Harpers Ferry beyond (signage along the trails makes finding these attractions a simple prospect).

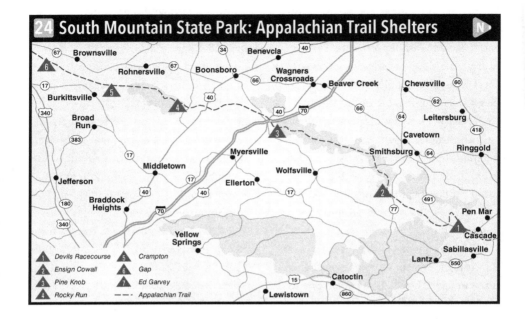

:: Getting There

From I-70 East: Take Exit 42, MD 17. Bear right onto MD 17 North. Turn left onto US 40 West and follow for just over 3 miles to the parking area before I-70. From I-70 West: Take Exit 35/MD 66. Bear right onto MD 66. Turn left onto US 40 East. Follow for 2.5 miles to the parking area on the right.

GPS COORDINATES
Rocky Run: N39°46094" W77°63087"
Crampton Gap: N39°41259" W77°63702"
Ed Garvey: N39°35982" W77°66172"
Trailhead: N39°32'08.7" W77°36'15.3"
Pine Knob: N39°54249" W77°60181"
Ensign Cowall: N39°63102" W77°55566"
Raven Rock: N39°673273" W77°52949"

25

South Mountain State Park:
Appalachian Trail Backpackers' Campgrounds

For AT thru-hikers, Dahlgren is a veritable paradise.

South **Mountain State Park** runs more than 8,000 acres, following the ridge of South Mountain from Pen Mar—just south of the Pennsylvania border—to Weverton, just north of the Potomac River. Total park acreage is 13,000 and includes South Mountain State Battle-field, site of the September 1862 Civil War battle. The park provides year-round access to the Appalachian Trail. The trail itself goes more than 2,000 miles from Maine to Georgia. Maryland's AT portion is 41 miles, running along the borders of Washington and Frederick Counties.

There are three backpackers' camp-grounds along the Maryland section of the AT: Dahlgren (something of a legend for AT thru-hikers), Pogo, and Annapolis

:: Ratings

BEAUTY: ★ ★ ★ ★
PRIVACY: ★ ★ ★
SPACIOUSNESS: ★ ★ ★
QUIET: ★ ★ ★
SECURITY: ★ ★ ★
CLEANLINESS: ★ ★ ★ ★

Rock. Using the Maryland AT midpoint overnight parking area off US 40, Pogo is 4 miles north, Annapolis Rock is 2.2 miles north, and Dahlgren is 5.2 miles south. The ratings below represent aver-ages for the three sites and will vary according to season; for instance, "pri-vacy" and "quiet" will skyrocket in winter and plummet in summer.

Officially there are 16 campsites at Pogo, but it's really one big area cleared for a dozen or more tents. A spring issues cold, clear water just a few feet from the trail. Often, privies at such primi-tive campgrounds like Pogo are situated between sites, but this one is up the hill, so if it emanates a bad smell, you should be far enough away that it won't bother you.

Closer to the parking area is Annapo-lis Rock. Campsites here are the newest of the three campgrounds, the result of a concerted effort from the Mary-land Department of Natural Resources, the AT Conference, and conservation-ists from the Virginia Polytechnic Insti-tute. Those who've camped at Annapolis Rock in the past have known some real

:: Key Information

ADDRESS: South Mountain State Park
c/o South Mountain Recreation Area
21843 National Pike
Boonsboro, MD 21713

CONTACT: South Mountain State Park:
301-791-4767, **dnr2.maryland.gov**;
Appalachian Trail NPS Park Office:
304-535-6278, **nps.gov/appa**

OPERATED BY: South Mountain State
Park is operated by the Maryland
Department of Natural Resources; the
Appalachian Trail is operated by the
National Park Service and a consor-
tium of local hiking and conservation
organizations.

OPEN: Year-round

SITES: 36+ (15 at Annapolis Rock [plus
3 group sites], 5+ at Dahlgren, 16 at
Pogo)

EACH SITE: Picnic table, fire ring (at
Pogo and Dahlgren), privy, water

ASSIGNMENT: First come, first served

REGISTRATION: None

FACILITIES: Showers at Dahlgren;
water shut off March–December

PARKING: None

FEE: Free

RESTRICTIONS

■ **Pets:** Permitted on a leash

■ **Quiet Hours:** Officially none, but
loud music and noises are discouraged.

■ **Visitors:** The Appalachian Trail Conservancy suggests hiking and camping in groups no larger than 10
people. Larger groups will be directed
away from Annapolis Rock.

■ **Fires:** In fire rings only (no fires at
Annapolis Rock)

■ **Alcohol:** Not permitted

■ **Stay Limit:** Practice and hikers'
etiquette dictate short stays of 1–2
days during warmer months, when
demand is highest.

■ **Other:** Limit visits on weekends, holidays, and during peak fall foliage.

ambivalence about the experience. Its namesake attraction is obvious: an outstanding perch above beautiful rolling and forested mountains. (Sunsets and sunrises here are magical.) But the refrain in describing Annapolis Rock over the years has been that it's "loved to death." Legions of campers stripped the area of wood, the soil had been made barren by a multitude of fires, and trash was an ever-present problem.

About a decade ago, work crews constructed campsites in a thickly vegetated area, away from the rock cliff. The following spring, they revegetated the denuded area. The resulting site, though still often crowded, is much improved, with 15 individual sites that hold up to 75 campers, two privies, and a caretaker to minimize harmful impact. Sites are built into the hillside to prevent erosion and are comparatively private.

The only campground south of the parking area, Dahlgren, is diminutive, with only five tent pads, each with a picnic table and a grill. However, there is a lot of cleared space between the trees and the tent pads, enough for dozens more tents,

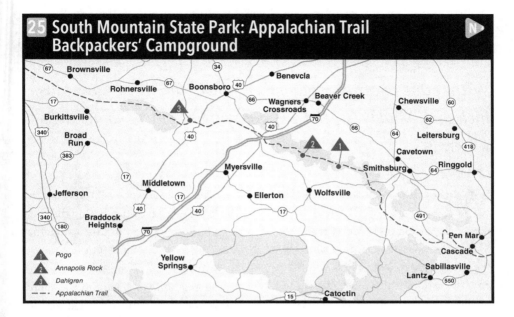

South Mountain State Park: Appalachian Trail Backpackers' Campground

which is the usual practice. For AT thru-hikers, Dahlgren is a veritable paradise because of its free hot showers, the only ones for some 2,000 miles of the AT. However, the hot water is shut off December to March. Two miles north of Dahlgren is Washington Monument State Park, home of the country's first monument to our first president, erected in 1827.

These three campsites sit within 10 miles of each other, so you can easily camp at each for successive nights without having to haul gear very far. Plus, the myriad side trails and numerous attractions in the area make this portion of the AT a truly wonderful place to hike and camp.

:: Getting There

From the east: On I-70, take Exit 42, MD 17. Bear right onto MD 17 North. Turn left onto US 40 West and follow it for just over 3 miles to the parking area before I-70. From the west: On I-70, take Exit 35, MD 66. Bear right onto MD 66. Turn left onto US 40 East. Follow for 2.5 miles to the parking area on the right.

GPS COORDINATES

Trailhead: N39°32'08.7" W77°36'15.3"

Annapolis Rock: N39°33' 38.97" W77°36' 2.07"

Dahlgren: N39°29' 0.47" W77°37' 9.07"

Pogo: N39°34' 31.31" W77°35' 5.34"

26

Swallow Falls State Park

Within this relatively small park, you'll find three waterfalls, including Muddy Creek Falls, Maryland's tallest single-drop waterfall.

Within this relatively small park (257 acres), you'll find three waterfalls (including Muddy Creek Falls, Maryland's tallest single-drop waterfall), the Youghiogheny Wild and Scenic River, and the oldest white pine and eastern hemlock in the state, with some trees approaching 400 years old. The park's name derives from the cliff swallows that used to nest on the rock pillar below the upper Swallow Falls. The area was drawing admirers long before it became a park. Some of the legends of American entrepreneurship (Ford, Firestone, and Edison, among them) camped along the falls, hoping for inspiration. Though your trip here won't be nearly as rugged, you can draw inspiration just the same within some spectacular scenery.

:: Ratings

BEAUTY: ★ ★ ★ ★ ★
PRIVACY: ★ ★ ★
SPACIOUSNESS: ★ ★
QUIET: ★ ★ ★
SECURITY: ★ ★ ★ ★ ★
CLEANLINESS: ★ ★ ★ ★ ★

The trail network near and around the falls can get crowded during the summer, but hiking here is a treat nonetheless. If you want more privacy (and a rugged hike), head for the 5-mile trail to Herrington Manor Park to the south, along a defunct tram road used for logging in the 1800s. The trail between the two parks takes in streams and hardwood forests home to a myriad of woodland creatures, including black bears and bobcats, among others.

There's fishing in the Youghiogheny too. Each year, the river is stocked with rainbow and brown trout. Native fish species include rock and smallmouth bass, chub, and white and northern hog sucker.

The majority of visitors to Swallow Falls will be day-trippers taking advantage of the easy trails running through hemlock forests and along the Youghiogheny River, where one can take in Muddy Creek, Upper Swallow, Lower Swallow, and Tolliver Falls. (Regrettably, major storms in 2015 did significant damage to the hemlocks lining the falls.) As a result, the park can get quite crowded during the day, but the campground—because it is reached

:: Key Information

ADDRESS: Swallow Falls State Park
2470 Maple Glade Road
Oakland, MD 21550

CONTACT: 301-387-6938;
dnr2.maryland.gov

OPERATED BY: Maryland Department
of Natural Resources

OPEN: Tolliver: late May–September;
Garrett: early April–mid-December

SITES: 65

EACH SITE: Fire ring, picnic table,
lantern post, tent pad

ASSIGNMENT: Tolliver: first come, first
served in May and September;
Garrett: first come, first served April–
May and October–mid-December

REGISTRATION: Reservations recommended late May through August;
888-432-2267 or **reservations.dnr**
.state.md.us

FACILITIES: Picnic area, pavilion, playground, bathhouse

PARKING: Maximum 2 vehicles/site

FEE: $21.49 plus service charge/night,
$32.49 plus service charge/night elec-
tric, water, and sewer; additional day-
use service charge during high season
$3–$5

RESTRICTIONS

▦ **Pets:** Allowed in the campground
but not permitted in the day-use area
from the Saturday before Memorial
Day–Labor Day

▦ **Quiet Hours:** 10 p.m.–7 a.m.

▦ **Visitors:** Maximum 6 people/site

▦ **Fires:** In fire ring only

▦ **Alcohol:** Permitted only inside
cabins and at shelters with valid
permit, as applicable

▦ **Stay Limit:** 2 weeks

▦ **Other:** 2-night minimum stay for
weekends, 3-night for holiday weekends. Check-in before 10 p.m.; checkout noon; Mid-October–December is
primitive camping. This is bear country;
take proper precautions.

by heading left when everyone else goes right—feels relatively secluded and peaceful. Your two camping choices are the Garrett Loop and the Tolliver Loop, which come after the youth group area (where you can access the 5-mile trail to Herrington Manor Park).

First up is Garrett Loop, with sites 1–5, 7, 33, 35, 37, and 39–64 (54, 56, and 58 are mini-cabins). Odd-numbered sites on the outside of the loop are usually preferable because they afford slightly more privacy. Sites 43 and 45 are the most isolated.

Tent-only sites in this loop are 46, 47, 49, 50, 51, 53, 61, and 62; of these, sites 49 and 51 are my favorites, as they have a bit of a drop-off on each side and sit near other tent-only sites. This is true only for these two, as all others will have at least one RV site as its neighbor (though the loop's only three electric sites—40, 42, and 42A—are generally farther away from all the tent sites except for 46). Two wheelchair-accessible sites, 4 and 60, are also available.

Tolliver Loop contains sites 6, 8, 9–32, 34, 36, and 38. Tolliver sits beyond Garrett

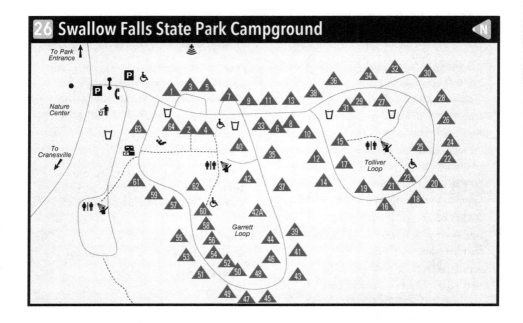

26 Swallow Falls State Park Campground

and so sees a bit less car traffic. It also has fewer sites total, which can be an advantage; however, all sites accommodate RVs. Of these, only 19, 21, and 23 are electric, so it's probably best to try and snag a site on the other end of the loop from these (they sit on the inner portion of the western edge of the loop). Sites 30, 32, and 34 are in a nice spot on the outer lower edge, across from the path to the bathhouse. If you require lots of room, sites 9, 11, 13, 15, and 27 are significantly larger than the others. Site 6 is the largest in all of Swallow Falls.

Sites are relatively small, without much space between them, but they are nicely wooded and pleasant nonetheless. Because of the limited number of sites, the campground doesn't feel packed. My slight preference, despite not being designated for tents only, is the Tolliver Loop, as most sites sit within pine and hemlock copses, which are exceedingly pleasant.

:: Getting There

Take I-68 to Exit 14, MD 219 South. Go 20 miles to Mayhew Inn Road and turn right. At the stop sign at the end of the road, turn left onto Oakland Sang Run Road. Take the first right onto Swallow Falls Road.

GPS COORDINATES N39°29'48" W79°25'31"

27

Youghiogheny River Lake:
Mill Run Campground

After its spectacular Class IV–V rapids in Maryland,
the Youghiogheny River is dammed, producing the recreational
haven of Youghiogheny River Lake.

Most people in the tri-state area (Maryland, Pennsylvania, and West Virginia) regard Youghiogheny River Lake as a Pennsylvania possession. Indeed, though the lake straddles the Mason–Dixon Line, the majority of it lies in Pennsylvania. Furthermore, the majority of whitewater rafting trips down the Youghiogheny commence from Pennsylvania locations: Ohiopyle and Confluence, to be precise (though real whitewater aficionados head for the Upper Yough, from Sang Run to Friendsville, in Maryland).

The river flows northward and, after its spectacular Class IV–V rapids in Maryland, it's dammed, producing the recreational haven of Youghiogheny River Lake. The U.S. Army Corps of Engineers maintains three campsites along the lake; two of them (Outflow and Tub Run) sit in Pennsylvania. They are the larger two of the three and are worth a visit. You can contact Outflow by calling 877-444-6777 or go to **recreation.gov.** For Tub Run, contact the Laurel Highlands Outdoor Center at **laurelhighlands.com/yough-lake-campground-tub-run** or call 800-472-3846. Here I'll concentrate solely on Youghiogheny River Lake's only Maryland campsite: Mill Run.

Despite containing a boat launch for the lake, the campground feels nicely isolated, partly due to the fact that it's located in a sparsely populated area of the state. Additionally, Mill Run Campground sits in a woodsy copse adjoining the Mill Run, a tributary of the Youghiogheny. Because the other two campgrounds on the lake are significantly larger and more popular, Mill Run can

:: Ratings

BEAUTY: ★ ★ ★ ★ ★
PRIVACY: ★ ★
QUIET: ★ ★ ★ ★
SPACIOUSNESS: ★ ★ ★
SECURITY: ★ ★ ★ ★ ★
CLEANLINESS: ★ ★ ★ ★

:: Key Information

ADDRESS: Mill Run Recreation Area Friendsville, MD 21531

CONTACT: 814- 395-3242

OPERATED BY: U.S. Army Corps of Engineers

OPEN: Year-round (reduced facilities mid-September–April)

SITES: 30

EACH SITE: Table and fire ring

ASSIGNMENT: First come, first served

REGISTRATION: Self-registration May–mid-September; no registration required otherwise

FACILITIES: Restrooms (no showers), playground, dump station, drinking water, phone, swimming beach, boat launch

PARKING: Vehicles not allowed on grass; multiple units allowed at each campsite so long as they fit within the boundaries of the site

FEE: When self-registration is in effect: $15/night; pay by check to Army Corps of Engineers, Pittsburgh; free mid-September–end of April

RESTRICTIONS

■ **Pets:** Must be leashed or caged

■ **Quiet Hours:** 10 p.m.–6 a.m.

■ **Visitors:** Maximum 6 people/site; guests must leave by 10 p.m.

■ **Fires:** In fire rings

■ **Alcohol:** Not permitted

■ **Stay Limit:** 2-week limit within 30 days

■ **Other:** Checkout 4 p.m.

feel like paradise found. This is not to say that you shouldn't expect company during the day, especially in summer.

If you're a boater, take advantage of what is widely considered the best boating and waterskiing lake anywhere near. If you've brought along the fishing pole, angle for walleye, bass, and trout. And, of course, there's always the whitewater rafting. After West Virginia's Gauley River, the Yough is arguably the East's best whitewater rafting locale.

Beyond the lake itself, recreational activities abound to the south. The Youghiogheny Scenic and Wild River was named as such in 1976, becoming Maryland's first river with such a designation.

A 21-mile stretch from Friendsville to Oakland remains protected and thrives as a beautiful and clean river even though it retains its popularity as a whitewater rafting hot spot. (For recreational opportunities on the Youghiogheny Scenic and Wild River, visit **dnr2.maryland.gov/public lands/Pages/western/youghiogheny .aspx** or call 301-387-5563.) As for the campground itself, it is a bit rustic, to put it nicely. Scoffers will call it run-down. I would call it a great place to stay for cheap that offers access to the lake. Some of the sites (15–18) are spitting distance from the boat ramp, with site 18 being the closest. The first few sites (1–8) are near the campground entrance and are not terribly

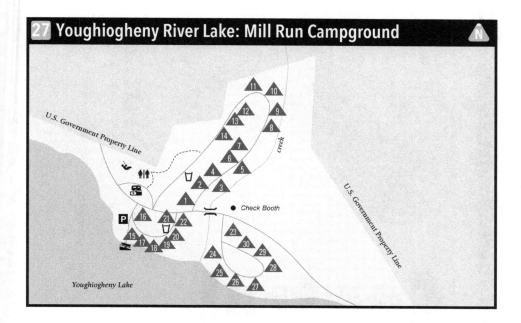

special. They sit right next to one another. But the farther you move to the right, the more private the sites get, with site 11 being the best in terms of privacy. My favorite sites in the campground are those down the hill across from the camp host, numbered 23–30. The most private ones are 26 and 27, as they sit on the farthest edge of the campground.

Remember, if you want to be in the center of all the action around Yough River Lake, head for the Pennsylvania campsites. (From Mill Run, if you continue up Friendsville-Addison Road and then go left at Addison, you'll get to the main recreation areas of the lake.) Mill Run is a bit away from it all, but this can be a good thing.

:: Getting There

Take I-68 to Exit 4, MD 53 North, Friendsville-Addison Road. Go through Friendsville and look for the signs to Mill Run to the left around 5.5 miles from town. The campground will be in a few miles at the end of the road.

GPS COORDINATES N39°42'55.4" W79°23'04.4"

Central Maryland

28

Cedarville State Forest

Spring is a fantastic time to visit Cedarville, as the wildflowers that dot the swamplands explode in color.

It pains me now, but I grew up within an hour of Cedarville State Forest (3,510 acres) and have become familiar with it only recently, now that I live much farther away. But better late than never because it's a great place.

The Piscataway Indians knew this, choosing the area around Cedarville Forest as their winter camping ground. They were well adapted to the ecology of the area, which is adjacent to the largest freshwater swamp in the state, Zekiah Swamp, which is a mile wide in some places and drains into the Wicomico River, some 20 miles away. The park contains the Cedarville Bog, at the swamp headwaters, allowing for an environment Marylanders don't see so much of, as the atmosphere conjures something closer to the Southeast. Correspondingly, insect-eating plants, a relative rarity in Maryland, flourish here. Diamond-back terrapins, a state mascot, live within the swamp areas and their tributaries. Bald eagles also nest here. With more than 19 miles of trails in the forest, a hiker can cover them all in a few days and take in the forest's wonderful ecological treasures, including loblolly pine plantations, planted in the 1930s by the Civilian Conservation Corps. If all this forest and swampland isn't enough, there's also the 4-acre Cedarville Pond, stocked with bass, bluegill, catfish, and sunfish (a Maryland nontidal sportfishing license is required). The pond area, accessible from the Green and Brown Trails down the forest road and over Zekiah Swamp Run, is the best place to see the swamp environment. A managed forest conservation area hosts some 50 different tree species.

Spring is a fantastic time to come here, as the wildflowers that dot the swamplands explode in color. An abundance of wildlife thrives in the managed forest, while the swamp waters attract loads of beaver and birds.

:: Ratings

BEAUTY: ★ ★ ★ ★
PRIVACY: ★ ★ ★ ★
SPACIOUSNESS: ★ ★ ★
QUIET: ★ ★ ★ ★
SECURITY: ★ ★ ★ ★ ★
CLEANLINESS: ★ ★ ★ ★ ★

:: Key Information

ADDRESS: Southern Maryland Recreational Complex, Cedarville SF 10201 Bee Oak Road Brandywine, MD 20613

CONTACT: 301-888-1410; **dnr2.maryland.gov**

OPERATED BY: Maryland Department of Natural Resources

OPEN: Late March–October

SITES: 27, plus potential overflow equestrian sites

EACH SITE: Parking pad, picnic table, fire ring

ASSIGNMENT: Walk-in and reservable

REGISTRATION: 888-432-CAMP (2267) or **reservations.dnr.state.md.us**

FACILITIES: Bathhouse, pavilion, dump station

PARKING: 2 vehicles/site

FEE: $18.49 plus service charge/night, $24.49 plus service charge/night electric; additional day-use fee $3–$5

RESTRICTIONS

▓ **Pets:** Permitted on leash

▓ **Quiet Hours:** 11 p.m.–7 a.m.

▓ **Visitors:** Maximum 6 people and 2 tents/site

▓ **Fires:** In fire rings

▓ **Alcohol:** Permitted only inside cabins and at shelters with valid permit, as applicable

▓ **Stay Limit:** 2 weeks

▓ **Other:** 2-day minimum required Memorial Day–Labor Day

Cedarville State Forest has 27 campsites in one loop. Pass the youth group camping area for family camping. Of the 27 sites, 4 are walk-in (sites 1, 8, 24, and 27). For walk-in, just pick a spot marked available and drop your money in the envelope at the bulletin board. Site 2 is reserved for the camp host. Reservable sites include 3–7, 9–12, and 25–26. The electric sites are the even-numbered sites between 4 and 24; all of these sit on the internal section of the loop, which means you'll want to shoot for the external sites. Among those, the sites that sit farthest from the electric (RV) sites are 7, 1, 2, 3, 26, and 27, but it's better to avoid the ones closest to the entrance (1, 26, and 27), as the area can get busy with patrolling rangers. The only bathhouse,

which was nicely renovated in 2012, sits in the middle of the loop. Firewood can be purchased at the campground. Spring water is also available.

The campsites are well shaded and spaced. There's often 100 feet or more between sites. Many sites sit right across the road from one another (as opposed to staggered) and thus don't offer oodles of privacy. The camping area is very small, and it's easy to feel close to your neighbors. The sites on the outside of the loop seem to be the better ones, as they're slightly more private. Of these, I think 9, 11, 17, 19, 21, and 23 are the nicest.

A friendly park ranger explained to me that if the park is full (say, on a holiday weekend), they might open up the

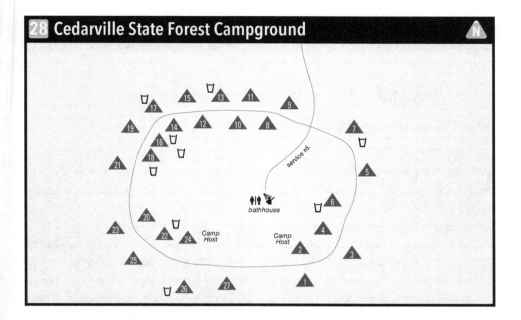

28 Cedarville State Forest Campground

primitive equestrian sites for family camping. Don't count on it, but it might be
worth asking. These sites are primitive but
much better shaded and much more private (all this assumes you don't mind seeing horse trailers).

:: Getting There

From I-495, take Exit 7A/MD 5 S/Branch Avenue toward Waldorf. Follow MD 5 south
10 miles to US 301 and continue south another 1.7 miles. Turn left at the stoplight
onto Cedarville Road (look for the state forest sign). In 2.3 miles turn right at Bee
Oak Road. The campground is in 1.9 miles.

GPS COORDINATES N38°39'0.7" W76°48'44.2"

29

Louise F. Cosca Regional Park

Cosca Regional Park is very much a family affair, with recreation galore.

Cosca Regional Park began in 1967 as Clinton Regional Park, Prince George's County's first regional park. A few years after its inception, its name was changed to honor the former Park and Planning Commissioner who saw it to its fruition. If she were around today, Ms. Cosca would no doubt be unhappy about the chockablock development just down Thrift Road from the park. But the park itself feels that much more like an oasis as a result.

Admittedly, I didn't have very high hopes on my first visit to Cosca. The park sits in Clinton, a populated D.C. suburb that no one would ever associate with good camping. But what a pleasant surprise awaited me. First, the park itself is very much a family affair, with recreation

:: Ratings

BEAUTY: ★ ★ ★
PRIVACY: ★ ★ ★
SPACIOUSNESS: ★ ★
QUIET: ★ ★ ★
SECURITY: ★ ★ ★ ★
CLEANLINESS: ★ ★ ★ ★

galore: ball fields, a tennis bubble, picnic areas, a lake and boathouse, a nature center, and much more. It's clearly a local favorite.

At 600 acres, the park is a decent size and offers more than 5 miles of trails for hiking or horseback riding. At the lake, folks can fish year-round and boat during the warmer months. The lake is stocked with bass, bluegill, catfish, and trout. The Clearwater Nature Center is truly a community affair, offering loads of nature programs geared toward kids and adults, and it's free, as is admission to the park itself. The center also hosts plenty of clubs to join.

What's especially nice is that the campground is across the road from the major sites listed above. As a result, it feels fairly secluded, though hiking trails easily link you to the rest of the park. The sites are wooded, with generally 50 feet or so between them. There's a picnic area, a playground, and a bathhouse in the camping area; generally speaking, everything is well maintained and clean. The bathhouse itself, however, is not in the best shape, to say the least. However, it is slated for an upgrade some time in 2016–17.

:: Key Information

ADDRESS: Cosca Regional Park
11000 Thrift Road, Clinton, MD 20735

CONTACT: 301-868-1397;
pgparks.com

OPERATED BY: Maryland-National
Capital Park and Planning Commission and Prince George's County
Department of Parks and Recreation

OPEN: Year-round

SITES: 25 (including 2 group sites)

EACH SITE: Picnic table, fire ring, tent pad

ASSIGNMENT: First come, first served

REGISTRATION: At the park office
(cash or check only)

FACILITIES: Picnic areas and shelters,
tennis courts, ball fields, boathouse,
playgrounds, comfort stations

PARKING: On paved areas only

FEE: Prince George's and Montgomery
County residents: $12/night, $15/night
electric ($10 and $13 for seniors); nonresidents, $20 and $23, respectively

RESTRICTIONS

▓ **Pets:** On a leash

▓ **Quiet Hours:** 10 p.m.–7 a.m.

▓ **Visitors:** No policy

▓ **Fires:** In fire rings only

▓ **Alcohol:** Not allowed

▓ **Stay Limit:** 2 weeks

▓ **Other:** Maximum 1 camping unit/
site

To get a site, head to the campground, pick whichever available one you like, then go to the park office and pay your fee. Avoid sites 8, 9, 11, and, to a lesser extent, 12; you can see houses through the trees behind these sites—the best way to spoil the illusion of sleeping out in nature. Sites 8 and 9 are reserved for groups of 15–30 people in any case.

Site 13 is nice, as it sits by itself. Site 14 is also good and secluded, and 1–7 are decent; site 3 might be an exception to this, as it sits closest to the bathhouse and small playground. Site 15 has the drawback of not being very level. Sites 16–22 seem to be the best; of these, 17 and 22 are my favorites. Site 16 has two picnic tables and pump water and is pretty spacious. Site 18 is also big; for this site, you pull into the parking area, and the tent site is off to the left another 10 yards or so deeper in the woods.

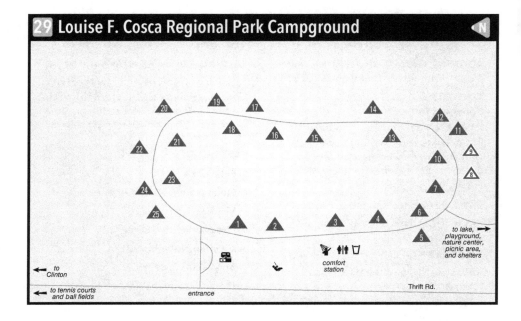

:: Getting There

Take I-495 to Exit 7A South/Branch Avenue/MD 5 toward Waldorf. Head south on Branch Avenue. After 4.3 miles, make a right onto Woodyard Road. At 0.7 mile, turn left onto Brandywine Road. In 1 mile, take a right onto Thrift Road, and go 1.3 miles. The campground will be on your right.

GPS COORDINATES N38°44'10.5" W76°54'37.6"

30

Elk Neck State Park

Visitors consistently remark how amazingly clean this park is.

Situated on a peninsula between the Chesapeake Bay and the Elk River, Elk Neck State Park contains a wealth of beauty (though no elk), encapsulated within a real diversity in topography, including beaches, marshes, and forests. Despite this, even on busy weekends, there's almost always a spot to stay, so you can feel comfortable making a last-minute decision to go and get a walk-in site. That said, much of this has to do with its size, as there are more than 250 sites. This is a beloved and extremely popular park and increasingly accommodating to RVs and those with pets. (In fact, only 4 of the 258 sites are tent-only: 183, 184, 185, and 196 in the Bohemia Loop.) Another reason is its location, drawing folks from Baltimore, Philadelphia, and Delaware.

:: Ratings

BEAUTY: ★ ★ ★ ★
PRIVACY: ★ ★
SPACIOUSNESS: ★ ★
QUIET: ★ ★ ★
SECURITY: ★ ★ ★ ★ ★
CLEANLINESS: ★ ★ ★ ★ ★

Expect crowds and not much privacy. Still, it's difficult to spend a few days at Elk Neck and not have a pleasant experience. Fishing, birding, hiking, boating, and swimming are popular activities.

Visitors consistently remark how amazingly clean this park is. Considering the heavy usage, it's a real testament to the staff. While it may be difficult to achieve total privacy at a popular park like Elk Neck, essentially every loop sits near a hiking trail or the water, so it's not difficult to escape, and the scenery never fails to impress.

Turkey Point Road (MD 272) is the main road that splits the park and ends at the parking area for the popular Blue Trail with its main attraction, the Turkey Point Lighthouse. The highest of the Chesapeake Bay's 74 lighthouses, it was built in 1833. But before you get there, you'll turn left on Campground Access Road. From there, you can reach any of Elk Neck's 12 camping loops (though some are for youth groups and some contain cabins). After passing the registration booth, if you take the first right, you'll come first to the North East Loop, which contains 31 sites, all with full hookups for RVs.

:: Key Information

ADDRESS: Elk Neck State Park
4395 Turkey Point Road
North East, MD 21901

CONTACT: 410-287-5333;
dnr2.maryland.gov

OPERATED BY: Maryland Department
of Natural Resources

OPEN: Year-round in Chester and
North East Loops; late March–Sept. in
Elk Loop; mid-March–late October in
Elk and Miles Loops; mid April–early
September in Bohemia, Wye, and
Susquehanna Loops; mid-March to
early October in Choptank Loop.

SITES: 258

EACH SITE: Fire ring, picnic table, tent
pad

ASSIGNMENT: Reservable and walk-in

REGISTRATION: 888-432-CAMP,
reservations.dnr.state.md.us, or
walk-in at the ranger station on
Campground Access Road

FACILITIES: Boat launch, cabins, camp
store, dump station, playground, shelters, swimming beach, visitor center

PARKING: 2 vehicles/site

FEE: $21.49 plus service charge/night,
$27.49 plus service charge/night electric, $36.49 plus service charge/night
water and sewer; day-use fee $3-$5;
boat launch $10/vehicle; out-of-state
residents add $2

RESTRICTIONS

▧ **Pets:** Leashed pets allowed in North
East, Wye, Susquehanna, St. Martins,
Elk, Miles, and Choptank Loops

▧ **Quiet Hours:** 11 p.m.–7 a.m.

▧ **Visitors:** 6 people, 2 tents/site ($3/
person over maximum)

▧ **Fires:** In fire rings

▧ **Alcohol:** Permitted only inside
cabins and at shelters with valid
permit, as applicable

▧ **Stay Limit:** 2 weeks

Pass North East and you'll eventually come to five more loops. First up to the right are the Wye Loop and the Susquehanna Loop. Wye contains sites 32–61, and Susquehanna has sites 62–75. Both accommodate RVs, but neither has electrical hookups. Continuing on to the end of the road, you'll run into the three remaining loops: Choptank to the left, Elk to the right, and Miles straight ahead. But before you do, take note of St. Martins (76–80), a diminutive section with five spots. These are tent-only but are used for overflow and are not reservable.

Choptank (sites 91–121) sits closest to the White Trail, an interpretive foliage trail across from the large camp store. The entrance to Elk Loop (sites 122–151) is close to a playground (especially sites 122–124), but its southern edge (sites 136–139) is near Stony Point and Rogues Harbor and allows easy access for a vigorous trek through forest, beach, and marsh on the Orange Trail.

Last in this bunch is the Miles Loop (sites 152–181), closest of all to Stony Point and its attendant views over the mighty Elk River. If you do stay in Miles Loop, try to snag sites 162, 163, or 165, as they are nearest the water.

Your other option for camping is northeast of the loops described above. Take the same Campground Access Road, but this time pass the registration booth and keep going straight, past the playground and camp store (which has laundry, by the way). Then you can either go left for Chester and Bohemia loops or right for the Sassafras Loop. The youth group area sits beyond Sassafras at the end of the road.

Sassafras Loop (249–278) sits adjacent to an open field, which can be a pleasant way to camp, often overlooked by people who assume the more woods the better. Sites 249–257 all sit at the edge of the road, with the open field behind. The better sites are those farther out,

258–277. Note that the youth group area, and its potential for noise, is just down the road beyond the end of the loop.

Bohemia (sites 182–210) is a circular loop near the beach areas north of Thackeray Point and allows easy access to the Green Trail, which winds along marsh and small lakes. If you camp in Bohemia, definitely try to get site 196, which is not just tent-only, but also sits right up the hill from the water.

Lastly, Chester Loop (sites 221–248) feels most crowded, with the sites near one another in a series of little roads running between the loop ends. All the sites in Chester have electrical hookups, so that might dissuade you as well. If you do wind up here, the best sites in this loop are sites 222 and 233, as they sit on the outside of the loop and near only one other site.

Note that renovations being undertaken in 2016 will affect sites (and reservations) in the Miles and Chester Loops.

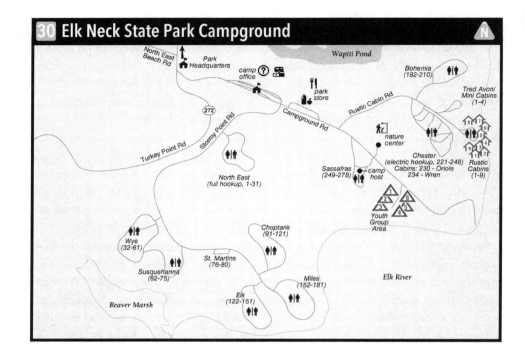

:: Getting There

Take I-95 from Baltimore to Exit 100/MD 272 S. Head south on MD 272 S, and go 9.8 miles. Turn right into the park.

GPS COORDINATES N39°30'10" W75°58'44"

31

Greenbelt Park

Your camp neighbor may very well be from across the country, or even across the globe.

When the federal government acquired land to build the Baltimore–Washington Parkway (Route 295) in 1950, Greenbelt Park (1,100 acres) was established as a sanctuary between the two big cities. It sits just 12 miles north of Washington and 23 miles south of Baltimore. Today, the corridor between Baltimore and Washington is highly developed, but Greenbelt Park remains a green sanctuary. According to the National Park Service, some 350,000 people visit the park annually, 20,000 of whom stay to camp. The result is that, depending on the season, you won't feel very alone or as if you're roughing it. However, the campground never fills up in the off-season and, amazingly, almost always has availability, even during cherry blossom time in the spring. A unique characteristic of

Greenbelt Park is that it functions as an inexpensive lodging alternative for visitors to D.C. Especially during the summer tourist season, your camp neighbor may very well be from across the country, or even across the globe, which can make for some interesting conversations.

The park's proximity to the capital is its chief attraction, but if you already live here, it is still a fine place to spend a few days. Wildlife isn't terribly exotic in the park, but it's abundant (my favorite are the foxes). A good place to spot wildlife, as well as enjoy some towering forest, is on the park's 6-mile Perimeter Trail. Aside from weaving through a deciduous forest, the trek also takes in three different creeks along the way. In all, there are some 9 miles of trails in the park.

Many visitors see the fact that the park is surrounded by major traffic arteries as a chief turn-off. But if you live in or near Central Maryland and need a quick escape, you couldn't ask for a better, more convenient choice. Additionally, the traffic noise isn't too bad. In fact, when I camped here in summer, the sounds of cicadas during the day and crickets at night effectively masked traffic noise.

:: Ratings

BEAUTY: ★ ★ ★
PRIVACY: ★ ★ ★
SPACIOUSNESS: ★ ★ ★
QUIET: ★ ★ ★
SECURITY: ★ ★ ★ ★ ★
CLEANLINESS: ★ ★ ★ ★ ★

:: Key Information

ADDRESS: Greenbelt Park
6565 Greenbelt Road
Greenbelt, MD 20770

CONTACT: 301-344-3948;
nps.gov/gree

OPERATED BY: National Park Service

OPEN: Year-round

SITES: 174

EACH SITE: Fire grate, picnic table

ASSIGNMENT: Reservable Memorial
Day–Labor Day; first come, first served
otherwise. If the office is closed, self-
register at the bulletin board just
beyond the park office.

REGISTRATION: 877-444-6777,
recreation.gov, or at park ranger station (open daily, 8 a.m.–3:45 p.m.)

FACILITIES: Restrooms, picnic tables,
water, fireplaces, utility sinks, dump
station

PARKING: Maximum 2 vehicles/site

FEE: $16/night ($8 for seniors holding
Golden Age Passes)

RESTRICTIONS

▓ **Pets:** Must be leashed

▓ **Quiet Hours:** 10 p.m.–6 a.m.

▓ **Visitors:** Maximum 6 people, 3
tents, and 2 vehicles/site

▓ **Fires:** In provided grills

▓ **Alcohol:** Prohibited

▓ **Stay Limit:** 14 days/year, limited to 7
days Memorial Day–Labor Day

▓ **Other:** Maximum 3 tents/site; checkout noon

Further, because there are no electrical hookups at any of the campsites, you
need not worry about RV electrical noise.

From Park Central Road, you'll
access the four camping loops: A (1–34), B
(35–83), C (84–110), and D (111–174). Skip
A entirely, as it is reserved only for Scouts.
In terms of noise, the best bet is probably
C, which sits the farthest from the major
roads that hem the park, though the difference in traffic noise between this loop
and the others is probably negligible.
Adding to the allure of Loop C, however, is the fact that it is tent-only. Aside
from this, most of the campsites in the
park are similar. The biggest difference
between them lies in the sites that have
long driveways for RVs (though, again, no
electrical hookups). Overall, the campsites are clean and well maintained.

All sites are wooded and nicely
shaded but without much room between
them. In some cases, it's barely 10 feet
from one campsite to the next. The most
you'll ever find between sites is around
75 feet. Nevertheless, most sites do back
up to thick woods, so while they all sit
very close to the campground roads and
neighbors, if you face your tent toward
the back of the site, you'll give yourself
the illusion of isolation.

I prefer Loop C because of its tent-
only status. This fact alone makes the
loop feel closest to camping in the woods.

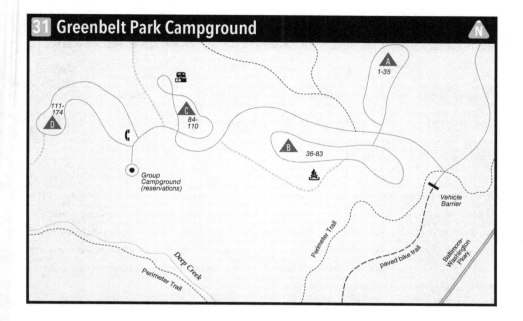

31 Greenbelt Park Campground

However, the most private sites I found are in Loop D. Site 119 feels pretty private, comparatively, and 174 is small but away from other campsites (though close to the campground road and the bathhouse). Sites 138–143 are open, in the middle of the camp loop, ideal for stargazing, though not very private. Sites on the outside of the loop, such as 147 and 149, tend to be the biggest and most private. Of these, 153 is decent.

In Loop B, sites 77 and 71 are nice, but my favorite is site 54, which sits down a little hill and feels most private. Also, because of a fallen pine, site 68 has a pleasant little natural barrier.

You're never too far from something at Greenbelt. Its proximity to the capital, its wooded sites, and its fine hiking trails are worth a visit.

:: Getting There

From I-495/I-95, take Exit 23/MD 201/Kenilworth Avenue. Head south on MD 201, and immediately take the exit for Greenbelt Road E/MD 193. Turn left onto Greenbelt, and the park is 0.25 mile down on the right.

GPS COORDINATES   N38°59'03.6" W76°53'45.3"

32

Hart-Miller Island State Park

If you want to fish, swim, and then pitch your tent under the stars and listen to the soft lap of small waves, you couldn't pick a better location.

If you want to feel like a modern-day Robinson Crusoe, take a boat to Hart-Miller Island State Park at the mouth of the Back River in the Chesapeake Bay. OK, it's not so remote that you'll feel like that famous castaway, but camping at Hart-Miller is a unique experience. Three islands comprise the park—Hart-Miller, Hawk Cove, and Pleasure Island—and each offers recreational activities and camping.

Some hiking trails exist on the islands, but they're few, and the park can be exhausted fairly easily. Hart-Miller Island is more than 1,100 acres in all, but much of it is off-limits, so don't expect oodles of recreation. Still, this isn't why people go to the island. If you've spent the day kayaking the area and want a place to stop, fish, swim, and then pitch your tent under the stars and listen to the soft lap of small waves, you couldn't pick a better location.

The U.S. Army Corps of Engineers began constructing Hart-Miller in 1981, using dredged materials from Baltimore Harbor and the channels leading to and from. Large wildlife restoration projects, some still ongoing, account for the disparity in size between the park and the larger island. Projects include re-creating forest, ponds, and habitat for migratory shorebirds, including wetlands and mudflats. Although the projects are still ongoing, Hart-Miller is already a place of major importance for migrating birds. Some 20,000 waterfowl have at times been seen on the island. Sandpipers and plovers share space with Caspian terns.

Don't be turned off by the fact that you must take a private boat to camp here. Getting to Hart-Miller is easy. The smallest of vessels—kayak or canoe is perfect—will get you there without a

:: Ratings

BEAUTY: ★ ★ ★ ★ ★
PRIVACY: ★ ★ ★ ★ ★
SPACIOUSNESS: ★ ★ ★ ★ ★
QUIET: ★ ★ ★ ★ ★
SECURITY: ★ ★
CLEANLINESS: ★ ★ ★ ★

:: Key Information

ADDRESS: Hart-Miller Island State Park
c/o Gunpowder Falls State Park
2813 Jerusalem Road
Kingsville, MD 21087

CONTACT: 410-592-2897;
dnr2.maryland.gov

OPERATED BY: Maryland Department
of Natural Resources

OPEN: Year-round; limited services
after October

SITES: 22 (6 on Hart-Miller, 11 at Hawk
Cove, and 5 on Pleasure Island)

EACH SITE: Primitive; there are picnic
tables and fire rings on the island

ASSIGNMENT: First come, first served

REGISTRATION: Rangers will collect
fee when they visit the island.

FACILITIES: Water and restrooms on
Hart-Miller at main camping area;
limited services after October

PARKING: None

FEE: $6/night

RESTRICTIONS

▓ **Pets:** Permitted on leash

▓ **Quiet Hours:** No official hours, but
rangers ask for courtesy toward all
visitors

▓ **Visitors:** Maximum 6 campers/site

▓ **Fires:** In fire rings

▓ **Alcohol:** Not permitted

▓ **Stay Limit:** None

▓ **Other:** Access only by private boat

problem. From the county-owned Rocky Point Beach and Park, the logical debarkation for Hart-Miller, it's less than 1.5 miles of easy paddling. This does, however, account for the low security rating above. I've never heard of any major problems at Hart-Miller, and neither had the ranger I spoke to, but the possibility exists of someone boating to the island and causing trouble. With no easy access back to land, the consequences could be serious. That said, don't let such a remote possibility dissuade you from camping at this unique spot, and be aware that rangers make frequent visits.

To get to Hart-Miller, park to the right just after the Rocky Point entrance. (Gates are open even after the park closes, and you can leave your car there overnight.) The ramp is at the end of the parking lot. Once in the water, swing around to the left; you'll pass North Point and then Pleasure Island. Hart-Miller is next. You'll see a mooring area as you approach to the right. A beautiful 3,000-foot beach tempts, and the primitive sites will soon come into view. Some are crudely marked, but the standing rule is that you can pitch your tent wherever there is space—and you can probably count on there being space.

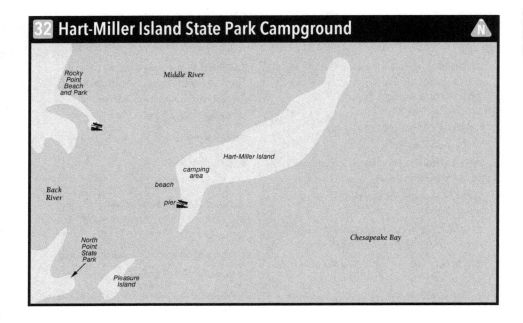

:: Getting There

To Rocky Point Beach and Park: Take I-695 to Exit 35/Southeast Boulevard/MD 702 S. Head south on MD 702, and travel 3.3 miles, where it turns into Back River Neck Road. In 2.4 miles, take a left onto Barrison Point Road and in 0.5 mile a right onto Rocky Point Road.

GPS COORDINATES N39°15'09.4" W76°22'24.4"

33

Little Bennett Regional Park

In a county that is increasingly suburbanized, this little slice of the natural world is cherished.

Little **Bennett Regional Park** has developed a loyal following among D.C.-area families looking for a quick and easy escape. Even the most extreme adventurer has to appreciate the 20-plus miles of trails within this 3,600-acre park that can be reached from either Baltimore or Washington in less than an hour.

The Hawk's Reach Activity Center serves as the park's center of activities, coordinating nature hikes, children's crafts, socials, and other family-geared entertainment. It also houses a popular game room. Large playgrounds, soccer fields, horseshoe pits, and volleyball courts provide additional entertainment and recreation for campers. I realize that the description above makes Little Bennett sound like a day camp swarming with

kids and burned-out adults. It's really much more pleasant than that; there's a sincere appreciation for the place that ripples through its users. In a county that is increasingly suburbanized, this little slice of the natural world is cherished. Several folks I spoke to described it as the perfect family camping spot—easy to get to and easy to love once you're there. The friendly staff ensures that it remains safe and full of activities. It's also extremely well maintained, with the sparkling-clean bathhouses being just one indication of that.

With so much wooded land within, Little Bennett manages to be quiet and serene, even with all the activity and recreation. In fact, hiking some of the outer trails can easily leave you feeling like the woods are yours alone. Additionally, the campsites are well wooded and nicely spaced.

Little Bennett's campsites are logically arranged, offering slightly different experiences for each loop depending on size and want. Loop A comes first, with sites 1–20, and it is tent-only. Preferable spots in Loop A include 13, 15, 17, 19, and 20. Loop A is also farthest from the electric loop. Slightly smaller Loop B contains

:: Ratings

BEAUTY: ★ ★ ★ ★
PRIVACY: ★ ★ ★
SPACIOUSNESS: ★ ★ ★ ★
QUIET: ★ ★ ★ ★
SECURITY: ★ ★ ★ ★ ★
CLEANLINESS: ★ ★ ★ ★ ★

:: Key Information

ADDRESS: Little Bennett Regional Park, 23705 Frederick Road Clarksburg, MD 20871

CONTACT: 301-528-3430; **montgomeryparks.org**

OPERATED BY: Maryland-National Capital Park and Planning Commission

OPEN: April 1–October 31; also open for weekend camping in March and November

SITES: 91

EACH SITE: Parking pad, picnic table, fire ring, lantern post, tent pad in 66 of the 91 sites

ASSIGNMENT: Reservations recommended, accepted after January 1 for any dates during that year's camping season

REGISTRATION: At **montgomeryparks .org**, 301-528-3430, or at the Contact Station: Sunday, 10 a.m.-6 p.m.; Monday–Thursday, 10 a.m.-7:30 p.m.; Saturday, 10 a.m.-8:30 p.m. (March and November: Tuesday and Friday, 8 a.m.-1 p.m.).

FACILITIES: Dump station, comfort stations, laundry room, activity and nature center, playgrounds, ball fields, camp store

PARKING: Maximum 2 vehicles/site

FEE: Military and seniors: $15–$35/ night; Prince George's and Montgomery County residents: $21–$41/night; nonresidents: $25–$49/night; hike-in sites (for up to 50 campers): $50/night

RESTRICTIONS

■ **Pets:** Permitted on leash and not left unattended

■ **Quiet Hours:** 11 p.m.–6 a.m.

■ **Visitors:** Maximum 6 people/site; visitors must register and pay at Contact Station

■ **Fires:** In fire ring

■ **Alcohol:** Not allowed

■ **Stay Limit:** 2 weeks

■ **Other:** Check-in noon; checkout 11 a.m.

sites 21–34 and is also tent-only; sites 30, 31, and 32 can be rented for $30–$35 a night as "camper-ready," meaning the staff at Little Bennett will have a four-person tent, two chairs, stove, and lantern all set up and waiting for you on arrival.

Loop C, also tent-only, is the most intimate of all, as it contains only 13 sites (35–47). Of these, 41, 43, and 45 are the nicest. Loop D, the park's only electric

loop, sits right across the road and contains sites 48–72.

Loop E, my favorite, contains sites 73–91. If you do stay in Loop E, note that sites 85 and 87 sit next to the Bennett Ridge Trail, which you can take to access the Beaver Valley Trail toward a beautiful spot at Little Bennett Creek. (There's an excellent trail map available at the Contact Station.) It might be nice to have that

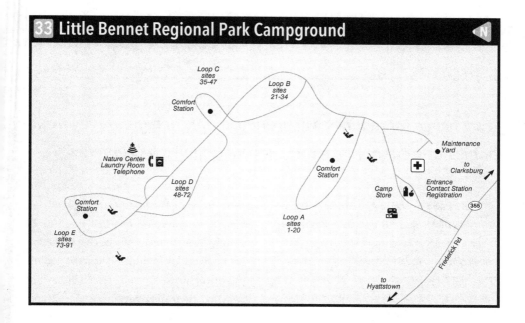

easy access, but be aware that you might also have close company by virtue of hikers accessing the trails. Sites 83 and 81 are also nice. If you have young kids with you, try for the internal sites on E: 74, 76, 78, 80, 82, 84, 86, 89, and 91. All give easy access to the playground in the loop without crossing the camp road.

:: Getting There

Take I-270 to Exit 18/MD 121/Clarksburg Road N. Head east on MD 121, and in 0.5 mile, take a left on MD 355/Frederick Road. The campground will be 1 mile ahead.

GPS COORDINATES N39°14'48.1" W77°17'27.1"

34

Patapsco Valley State Park:
Hilton Area

It's a haven for families who want a couple of nights away from home but want to reach their destination in a few minutes.

Patapsco Valley State Park **(PVSP),** straddling the Patapsco River and encompassing sections of four counties, can rightly be considered central Maryland's recreation granddaddy. Sprawling over 32 miles of the Patapsco River and encompassing 14,000 acres, PVSP possesses many miles of sublime hiking trails and an abundance of outdoor recreation activities within its five developed areas. Aside from its great reputation for hiking, PVSP offers fantastic fishing and mountain biking. Its location amid heavy population centers makes it a true haven for nature-seekers (many sections are entirely devoid of people and feel remote and wild). Those who haven't been to the park might never guess the beauty and solitude one can easily find simply by walking a mile or two (or less). It's a haven for families who want a couple of nights away from home but want to reach their destination in a few minutes. For these folks, even the occasional rumble of a train traversing the parkland is a small price to pay for the abundance of activities available and the ability to sleep safely in nature just a few miles from home.

I know PVSP primarily from hiking its many trails (more than 170 miles in all), and I used to be rather snobbish about regarding it as a camping destination: too busy, too crowded, and so on. However, I must admit to being pleasantly surprised the first time I visited the Hilton area's campground, and now, many years later, I regard it even more highly than I originally did. It's a true gem, far from the main action centers elsewhere in the park. It's also small and well wooded, assuring quiet and privacy that can be tough to get otherwise.

:: Ratings

BEAUTY: ★ ★ ★ ★
PRIVACY: ★ ★ ★ ★
SPACIOUSNESS: ★ ★ ★
QUIET: ★ ★ ★ ★
SECURITY: ★ ★ ★ ★ ★
CLEANLINESS: ★ ★ ★ ★ ★

:: Key Information

ADDRESS: Patapsco Valley State Park, 8020 Baltimore National Pike Ellicott City, MD 21043

CONTACT: 410-461-5005; **dnr2.maryland.gov**

OPERATED BY: Maryland Department of Natural Resources

OPEN: Late March–late October

SITES: 13, plus 6 mini-cabins

EACH SITE: Picnic table, fire ring, lantern post

ASSIGNMENT: Self-registration for walk-ins, but advance reservations recommended

REGISTRATION: 888-432-CAMP (2267) or **reservations.dnr.state.md.us**

FACILITIES: Playground, bathhouse, picnic area

PARKING: Only on camp pad, maximum 2 vehicles

FEE: $20/night

RESTRICTIONS

■ **Pets:** Not allowed

■ **Quiet Hours:** 10 p.m.–7 a.m.

■ **Visitors:** Must register and must leave by 9:30 p.m.; maximum 6 people/site

■ **Fires:** In fire rings

■ **Alcohol:** Permitted only inside cabins and at shelters with valid permit, as applicable

■ **Stay Limit:** 2-week maximum; 2-night minimum Memorial Day– Labor Day

■ **Other:** Check-in 3–10 p.m.

Hilton's chief attractions are its diminutive size and nonelectric status. Additionally, it sits near some great hiking trails. One of my favorites remains the yellow-blazed Buzzards Rock Trail. This stunning trail can be reached easily from the campground, which is surrounded by woods and more trails on all sides: Charcoal to the west, Santee Branch to the south and east (and accessed just within the campground entrance), and Sawmill Branch to the north. Sawmill Branch Trail ends at Buzzards Rock Trail, just before the stone CSX bridge and the paved Grist Mill Trail.

Buzzards Rock heads precipitously uphill and leads to (and then passes) the rock for which the trail is named. Buzzards used to congregate here because the site commands a view of the valley—and the prey lurking in the woods. It's spectacular, especially in the fall. Because it requires a hefty climb, I often have it to myself when I'm here. If you've brought your bike, the paved Grist Mill Trail follows the Patapsco River and eventually passes Lost Lake, a fishing lake reserved for those over age 61, those younger than age 16, or those with disabilities.

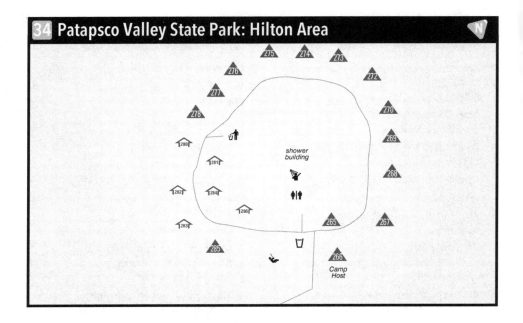

34 Patapsco Valley State Park: Hilton Area

Oddly, I find the Hilton campground often quite empty. I think locals see the Hilton area of PVSP mostly as a day-use area. Hilton has 13 tent-only campsites, plus one reserved for the camp host. Campers requiring heat and electricity can rent one of the six camper cabins, each recently outfitted with larger ceiling fans for cooling. To avoid the light coming from the cabins, choose sites farthest away; sites 277, 278,

and 285 are closest. Be aware that there's a power line cut behind sites 276 and 277, so they are a bit more open than the others, but even these are pleasant sites. Thick, mature trees surround all 13 sites, and all sit on the outside of the camp loop, while the bathhouse, always clean and well maintained, is on the inside. In my view, the best sites are 268, 269, 270, and 272. In short, this is a very pleasant campground.

:: Getting There

Take I-695 to Exit 13/Frederick Road toward Catonsville. Head west on Frederick Road, and go 1.2 miles to a left on S. Rolling Road. Go straight almost immediately at the big leftward curve onto Hilton Avenue. The park is 1.5 miles on the right.

GPS COORDINATES N39°14'50.8" W76°44'36.5"

35

Patapsco Valley State Park:
Hollofield Area

This park will keep kids (and their parents) happily entertained for days.

Despite its crowded feel (or maybe because of it), Patapsco Valley State Park (PVSP) is a logical camping destination for families, especially those with young kids. The reason is simple: If it doesn't work out for some reason, you can easily pack up and make the short trip home. Another attraction is that you can hop into the car and pick up any forgotten supplies in nearby towns.

When you enter the park's Hollofield area, you'll reach what many consider to be PVSP's epicenter. Within a short radius, you'll find a popular vista, playgrounds and picnic areas, hiking trails, and the park headquarters. The number of day-users here can get thick, and you

have to walk north to reach uncrowded trails. But once there, the Ole Ranger and Peaceful Pond Trails are fantastic, marked by sloping, wooded hills rising above the Patapsco River gorge. To enjoy all the features that make PVSP so attractive, you might find that you'll have to head south toward the Hilton, Avalon, Orange Grove, and Glen Artney areas. Once that easy trip is complete (and you can do it by floating down the river), there's a ton to do: boating, fishing, hiking, hunting, horseback riding, mountain biking, and nature and history programs put on by park rangers. In short, it is a place where kids (and their parents) can keep themselves happily entertained for days.

From the popular overlook, the campground is to the right, down the hill, and past the pavilions and boathouses. On the way to the campground, you'll pass the fabulous River Ridge Trail. One drawback to this day-use section is that it sits close to US 40, and road noise is pretty bad. But the campground is fairly far from the road; all you should hear is the occasional truck or motorcycle.

:: Ratings

BEAUTY: ★ ★ ★ ★
PRIVACY: ★ ★ ★
SPACIOUSNESS: ★ ★
QUIET: ★ ★ ★
SECURITY: ★ ★ ★ ★ ★
CLEANLINESS: ★ ★ ★ ★

:: Key Information

ADDRESS: Patapsco Valley State Park 8020 Baltimore National Pike Ellicott City, MD 21043

CONTACT: 410-461-5005; dnr2.maryland.gov

OPERATED BY: Maryland Department of Natural Resources

OPEN: Late March–late October

SITES: 73

EACH SITE: Camp pad, picnic table, fire ring

ASSIGNMENT: Reservations recommended, but same-day self-registration is allowed

REGISTRATION: If self-registering, go to camp headquarters, open Monday–Friday, 9 a.m.–3 p.m.; if no one is there, self-register by choosing available site and registering at the info desk. For reservations, call 888-432-CAMP (2267) or visit reservations.dnr.state.md.us.

FACILITIES: Bathhouses, camp store, playground, visitor center, frost-free spigot

PARKING: Only on camp pad, maximum 2 vehicles

FEE: $18.49 plus service charge/night, $24.49 plus service charge/night electric

RESTRICTIONS

▓ **Pets:** Allowed in all sites; must be leashed

▓ **Quiet Hours:** 10 p.m.–7 a.m.

▓ **Visitors:** Visitors must register and leave by 9:30 p.m.; maximum 6 people/site

▓ **Fires:** In fire rings

▓ **Alcohol:** Permitted only inside cabins and at shelters with valid permit, as applicable

▓ **Stay Limit:** Maximum 2 weeks

▓ **Other:** Check-in 3–10 p.m.; checkout 1 p.m.

Of PVSP's two campgrounds, Hollofield is the busier. It has 73 sites (400–472). In recent years, all sites in the entire campground have been made pet-friendly, assuming the dog is leashed and not left unattended for more than 30 minutes. The campground has two loops. One is diminutive, containing only sites 461–472, which are nonelectric, so this might be a good bet. The most private site in this loop is 469. A power line cut runs near sites 461 and 462, but there's a decent wooded buffer even here. There is no bathhouse in this loop.

All other sites sit north on one big loop. This is where you'll find the bathhouse (brand new as of 2016). In this loop, sites 406, 424, 425, and 430 are wheelchair accessible. Electric sites include 400–429, and tent-only are 430–460. I like site 454; 456 and 458 are good sites, too, but they are somewhat close to the loop's electric sites. The same power line cut that comes close to sites 461 and 462 in the other loop also cuts across the eastern section of this loop, coming closest to sites 432–436.

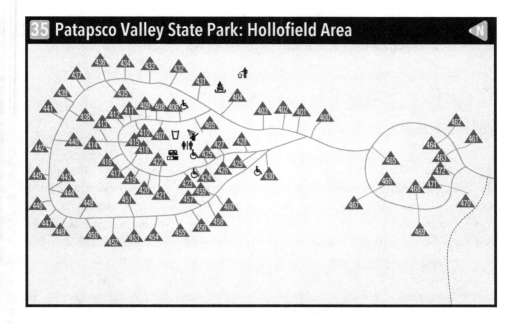

:: Getting There

Take I-695 to Exit 15B, US 40 W. Head west on US 40, and go 3 miles, and turn right into the park. (Once over the Patapsco River Bridge, the turn is in 0.4 mile.)

GPS COORDINATES   N39°17'43.6" W76°47'11.2"

36

Patuxent River Park

To say your space will be large is the understatement of the century.

Patuxent **River Park** comprises more than 6,000 acres of environmentally sensitive parkland along the eastern edge of Prince George's County, and it's an absolute jewel, doing a wonderful job of protecting a fragile natural treasure. Aside from the stunning natural area, the camping setup is a dream. There are six campsites total, but that number is misleading. Each site can accommodate more than two dozen campers; the park has hosted a couple of hundred campers before. (It's probably wise to ask if there are large groups scheduled to camp in the airfield. If so, ask for a spot far away.) But if you reserve a spot—even if you're camping alone—you get the site all to yourself. To say your space will be large, in that case, is the understatement of the century. Four campsites (A, B, C,

and D) are spread out along the edge of the defunct Croom Airfield, a large open field, and the distance between them is immense. If you're camping alongside 200 scouts, it might be unpleasant, but chances are just as good that you'll have a huge portion of the airfield to yourself. In either case, it's a bonus that no RVs or trailers are allowed.

Because there is so much space in the airfield, you can enjoy recreational activities in the area near your campsite. Your fee gives you access to a game room with basketballs, volleyballs, soccer balls, and horseshoes. There are 8 miles of trails for hikers and equestrians, as well as on-site museums. Additionally, the park supplies water and firewood.

As indicated above, there are four campsites in the airfield. Of these, D sits in a wooded copse. A and B are located along the edge of the woods on a little rise above the airfield. C is in the open, but woods border it on either side; depending on the time of day, this site can be shaded as well. Only D is consistently shaded, so if that's a priority, be sure to ask for it. I think it's great to be able to walk a little distance into the field and stargaze at night.

:: Ratings

BEAUTY: ★ ★ ★ ★
PRIVACY: ★ ★ ★ ★
SPACIOUSNESS: ★ ★ ★ ★ ★
QUIET: ★ ★ ★ ★
SECURITY: ★ ★ ★ ★ ★
CLEANLINESS: ★ ★ ★ ★ ★

:: Key Information

ADDRESS: Patuxent River Park, 16000 Croom Airport Road Upper Marlboro, MD 20772

CONTACT: 301-627-6074; **pgparks.com**

OPERATED BY: Maryland-National Capital Park and Planning Commission and Prince George's County Department of Parks and Recreation

OPEN: Year-round

SITES: 6

EACH SITE: Fire pit, firewood, picnic tables; some have toilets

ASSIGNMENT: Reservations required

REGISTRATION: 301-627-6074 (Tuesday–Friday, 8:30 a.m.–4 p.m.)

FACILITIES: Flush toilets, wildlife center, boat launch and rental, museums

PARKING: At the barn in the airfield, on site for canoe sites and Selby's campsites

FEE: Prince George's and Montgomery County residents: $20; nonresidents: $25

RESTRICTIONS

▨ **Pets:** Allowed

▨ **Quiet Hours:** None

▨ **Visitors:** Airfield, canoe, and Selby's campsites can accommodate up to 25

▨ **Fires:** In fire rings only

▨ **Alcohol:** Prohibited

▨ **Stay Limit:** None

▨ **Other:** Water must be obtained in the group camping site.

The two other sites, the canoe site and Selby's, both sit adjacent to Jug Bay; park literature calls Jug Bay "one of the most important freshwater tidal estuaries in the Chesapeake Bay region." Additionally, the Audubon Society has designated Jug Bay an Important Birding Area. More than 250 bird species have been spotted here, and more than 100 of these nest in the area. Of these two, I much prefer the canoe campsite, which is truly spectacular. Imagine a wooded campsite with your own personal road (a locked gate on the entrance road and you holding the key) and Jug Bay just 50 yards away from your spot. It's a camper's dream. Just beyond the gate, there's a big open parking area, flanking two toilets to the left. A buffer of foliage is next, and Jug Bay sits just beyond that. A little pier juts into the water, where you can launch and fish. Trails wind along the river's edge. Up a small rise to the right, within a thick stand of trees, is the camp area. Picnic tables and a grill are scattered among several level tent spaces. You can bring your own canoe or rent one here. The park even offers guided trips. Admittedly, the site is tough to get on weekends, but it's often free during the week. If you can reserve a few months in advance, your chances of getting it for

36 Patuxent River Park Campground

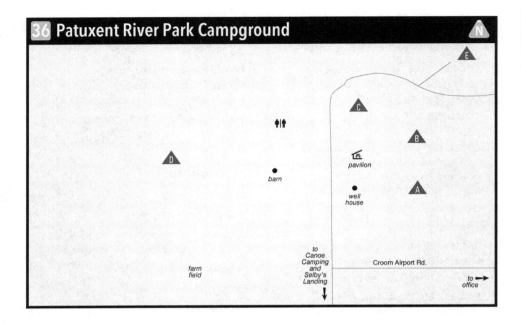

E

C

B

♦♦

pavilion

D

barn

well
house

A

to
Canoe
Camping
and
Selby's
Landing

Croom Airport Rd.

farm
field

to ➤
office

a weekend are decent. Obviously, most campers at Patuxent River Park wind up in the airfield, but if you can get the canoe spot, don't hesitate.

The site at Selby's Landing is a matter of personal taste. Because it's just to the right of the boat launch area, it's in the middle of all the action. Some people like this about Selby's, while others hate it for this same reason. The choice, of course, is up to you. To reach it, follow Croom Airport Road around the airfield until it ends.

:: Getting There

Take I-495 to Exit 11A for MD 4 S/Pennsylvania Avenue toward Upper Marlboro. Head south on MD 4/Pennsylvania Avenue, and go 7.5 miles. Take the US 301 exit toward Richmond, Virginia. Head south on US 301, and go 3.5 miles. Turn left on MD 382 (Croom Road) and go 3 miles. Turn left onto Croom Airport Road and travel 1.9 miles to the park.

GPS COORDINATES N38°45'12.6" W76°42'36.5"

37

Patuxent Water Trail

All sites are paddle-in only, which makes them unique and wonderful.

The **Patuxent Water Trail** is run by a consortium of environmental organizations dedicated to preserving the Patuxent River, which runs more than 100 miles through several central and southern Maryland counties before emptying into the Chesapeake Bay. (The Patuxent is the longest river entirely within the state.) There are five separate campsites along the river, four in Prince George's County and one in Charles County, in the more southerly portions of the Patuxent, where it approaches the bay. Each site is similar in that they are all, obviously, astride the Patuxent. They vary in the amount and kind of foliage and whether the pull-in area is marshy or sandy, but each is lovely and promises to please. (Of course, be prepared for bugs that like to hang out near water, including relentless summertime mosquitos.)

:: Ratings

BEAUTY: ★ ★ ★ ★ ★
PRIVACY: ★ ★ ★ ★ ★
SPACIOUSNESS: ★ ★ ★ ★
QUIET: ★ ★ ★ ★ ★
SECURITY: ★ ★ ★
CLEANLINESS: ★ ★ ★ ★ ★

To give a sense of distances and accessibility, note that each site below has a corresponding mile marker, running south–north in ascending order, beginning about 2.5 miles south of the Governor Thomas Johnson Bridge on the southern end of the Patuxent before it reaches the Chesapeake Bay, bridging the towns of California (St. Mary's County) and Solomons (Calvert County).

Note also that Nottingham Patuxent Riverkeeper Center in Upper Marlboro is located at mile marker 37; you can drive to it and park and launch from there for $5 (if you are a member of the organization, the launch is free). A nice visitor center is there as well. The contact number is 301-579-2073. You can even rent kayaks there by calling 855-725-2925 or e-mailing info@paxriverkeeper.org.

Running north to south, the first site is at Iron Pot Landing at mile marker 45. The closest launch site to the north is at Patuxent Wetlands Park (mile marker 47) in Lothian. To get there from I-495, take Exit 11A, and head south on MD 4/Pennsylvania Avenue. Turn left on MD 408/Mt. Zion Marlboro Road, and turn left and then left again onto the access road just after the MD 4 entrance ramp;

:: Key Information

ADDRESS: Varies (see text)

OPERATED BY: Maryland-National Capital Park and Planning Commission, Prince George's County Department of Parks and Recreation, Maryland Department of Natural Resources, Charles County Department of Parks

CONTACT: 301-627-6074; **patuxentwatertrail.org**

OPEN: Year-round

SITES: 5

EACH SITE: Picnic table, fire ring, portable toilet

ASSIGNMENT: First come, first served

REGISTRATION: Call Patuxent State Park at 301-627-6074.

FACILITIES: None

PARKING: None

FEE: Residents: $20/night; nonresidents: $24/night; no charge for Maxwell Hall

RESTRICTIONS:

- **Pets:** No restrictions
- **Quiet Hours:** None
- **Visitors:** Maximum 20 people/site
- **Fires:** In fire rings
- **Alcohol:** Permitted
- **Stay Limit:** None

go to the end of the road. To the south, launch at Patuxent River Park (mile marker 42; see page 134 for info).

Next up is White Oak Landing at mile marker 39. There is a decent amount of shade at White Oak, which isn't always the case with all the water trail sites. Nearest launch sites: From the north, use Selby's Landing (mile marker 40) at the Jug Bay Natural Area of Patuxent River Park (see page 134). From the south, use the Clyde Watson Boating Area at mile marker 31. To get to Clyde Watson, take I-495 to Exit 7A, and head south on MD 5. In 9 miles turn left onto Brandywine Road and continue on MD 381. In 9.8 miles turn left on MD 382/Croom Road. Go 2.2 miles and turn right onto Magruder's Ferry Road. Go 1.2 miles to park. (Also note that the Riverkeeper Center sits at mile marker 37; see previous page.)

The third site is at Spice Creek (mile marker 35); in my opinion, it's one of the nicest—a really beautiful little spot. The nearest launch sites are the Clyde Watson Boating Area to the south at mile marker 31 and Selby's Landing at mile marker 39 to the north. (For directions to both, see White Oak above.)

The next site is at Mill Town Landing (mile marker 30), a nice spot with a sandy spit to pull in. Launch sites sit just 1 mile north (Clyde Watson—see above) and 1 mile south (Kings Landing Park, in Huntingtown). To reach Kings Landing, from Exit 11A on I-495, head south on MD 4 to MD 262/Lower Marlboro Road. In 1 mile turn left onto Huntingtown Road and follow it 2.7 miles. Turn right onto Kings Landing Road and follow it until it ends.

The final campsite, in Charles County, is found at Maxwell Hall Park.

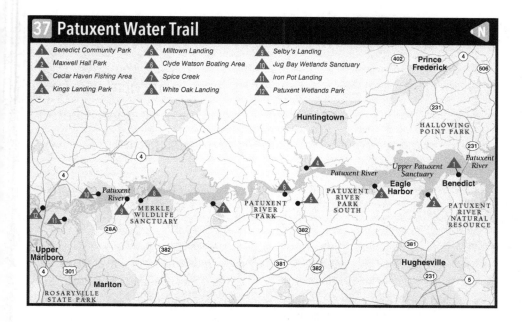

37 Patuxent Water Trail

1. Benedict Community Park
2. Maxwell Hall Park
3. Cedar Haven Fishing Area
4. Kings Landing Park
5. Milltown Landing
6. Clyde Watson Boating Area
7. Spice Creek
8. White Oak Landing
9. Selby's Landing
10. Jug Bay Wetlands Sanctuary
11. Iron Pot Landing
12. Patuxent Wetlands Park

There is no fee for using the site at Maxwell Hall. The nearest launch site to the north is Cedar Haven fishing area (mile marker 26) in Eagle Harbor. To reach Cedar Haven, take I-495 to Exit 7A, and head south on MD 5. In 9 miles turn left onto Brandywine Road and continue on MD 381. In 13.2 miles turn left onto Eagle Harbor Road. Travel 2 miles and bear left onto Trueman Point Road. Go 0.6 mile and bear left onto Banneker Boulevard. After 0.5 mile, the park entrance will be straight ahead. Benedict Community Park (mile marker 22) in Benedict is the nearest launch site to the south. Take MD 5 to MD 231 east to the Patuxent.

:: Getting There

Varies; see text.

GPS COORDINATES
Iron Pot Landing: N38°47'45" W76°43'14"
White Oak Landing: N38°44'33" W76°42'07"
Spice Creek: N38°41'34" W76°42'16"
Mill Town Landing: N39°37'58" W76°41'38"
Maxwell Hall: N38°31'49.5" W76°40'44"

38

Susquehanna State Park

John Smith's 1608 assessment of the area is applicable even today: "Heaven and earth seemed never to have agreed better to frame a place for man's . . . delightful habitation."

John **Smith first explored** the Susquehanna in 1608. Of course, the native Susquehannock Indians had already been hunting and fishing in the area for centuries. Smith's assessment of the area is applicable even today: "Heaven and earth seemed never to have agreed better to frame a place for man's . . . delightful habitation." True enough, if any local outdoor enthusiast needs a reminder why he or she is lucky to live in this area, Susquehanna State Park provides it. Among the Susquehanna River's impressive numbers: It's 444 miles long, includes a 13-million-acre drainage basin pouring 19 million gallons of freshwater into the Chesapeake Bay every minute, and it's the second largest watershed in the eastern United States.

:: Ratings

BEAUTY: ★ ★ ★ ★ ★
PRIVACY: ★ ★ ★
SPACIOUSNESS: ★ ★ ★
QUIET: ★ ★ ★
SECURITY: ★ ★ ★ ★ ★
CLEANLINESS: ★ ★ ★ ★ ★

A major draw for Susquehanna State Park is fishing. Striped, smallmouth, and largemouth bass are abundant. Anglers also catch channel catfish, carp, alewife, pike, and perch. This means that folks camping are often up and out early, especially in springtime during the annual herring and shad runs. If that's your primary motivation, too, don't worry. The river is large, and you can easily claim a prime spot. If your motivation for visiting Susquehanna State Park is hiking, be thrilled. The trails, more than 15 miles worth in all, can be surprisingly empty. One of them heads to the Conowingo Dam, a prime spot for birding. There's also much here in the way of historical attractions: The Rock Run Historic Area includes the still-operational Rock Run Grist Mill (1794), as well as the Rock Run Mansion (1804). There's also the Stepping-stone Museum, which includes antique farm implements, a restored farmhouse, decoy carving, and a blacksmith shop.

The campground contains two loops: Acorn (36–69) and Beechnut (1–35). Acorn is where you'll find the electrical

:: Key Information

ADDRESS: Susquehanna State Park
4122 Wilkinson Road
Havre de Grace, MD 21078

CONTACT: 410-557-7994;
dnr2.maryland.gov

OPERATED BY: Maryland Department
of Natural Resources

OPEN: Late March–late October

SITES: 71 (including 6 camper cabins)

EACH SITE: Picnic table, fire pit,
lantern hook

ASSIGNMENT: Reservations recommended, but if camping without,
check reservation board posted at the
campground entrance for availability.

REGISTRATION: 888-432-2267 or
reservations.dnr.state.md.us

FACILITIES: Bathhouse, water, boat
launch, playground, picnic areas, pavilions, bow-hunting area, archery range

PARKING: On gravel driveway

FEE: $21.49 plus service charge/night;
$27.49 plus service charge/night electric; day-use fee $3-$4; boat launch
$10/vehicle, $12 out-of-state residents

RESTRICTIONS

■ **Pets:** Must be leashed

■ **Quiet Hours:** 11 p.m.–7 a.m.

■ **Visitors:** 6 people, 2 tents/site
($3/person over maximum)

■ **Fires:** In fire rings

■ **Alcohol:** Permitted only inside
cabins and at shelters with valid
permit, as applicable

■ **Stay Limit:** 2-day minimum Memorial Day–Labor Day on weekends

■ **Other:** A Chesapeake Bay Sports
Fishing License (tidal license) is
required to fish the Susquehanna from
Conowingo Dam to the Chesapeake.

sites (38–43, 57, and 60). To best avoid these (as well as the light from the camper cabins), go for the sites on the outside upper edge of the loop: 48–53. Of these, site 52 is a terrific one, very private and nice. Generally speaking, the campsites are all pretty private and well spaced, so it's tough to find a bad spot in the Acorn Loop. Still, my favorite in Acorn is definitely site 59, which requires a hike-in of about 250 feet, making it comparatively private despite being near the electrical sites. If you can get this site, take it. The tent-only sites in Acorn are 50, 58, 59, 61–63, and 65–67.

Sites in the Beechnut Loop are not much different from Acorn, but the entire loop is nonelectric, so it might be preferable (only three sites, however—3, 24, and 26—are tent-only). If you do go there, consider park staff recommendations of sites 5, 10, and 18—these nice sites all guarantee a decent amount of privacy. Beechnut seems to be the more rugged and remote-feeling of the two loops, perhaps owing to its nonelectric status; however, as noted, relatively little else distinguishes one from the other. Both loops feature nice, newly renovated bathhouses.

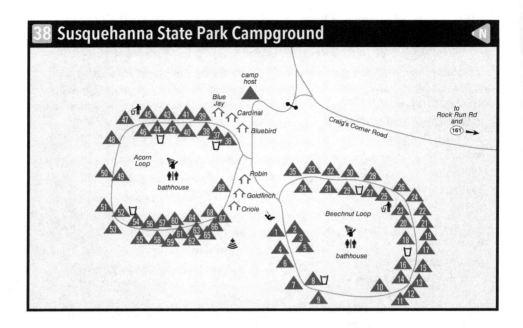

:: Getting There

Take I-95 to Exit 89/MD 155 W. Head west on MD 155, and go 2.9 miles. Turn right on MD 161. Go 0.3 mile and turn right on Rock Run Road. Follow Rock Run into the park. Follow signs to the camping area.

GPS COORDINATES   N39°36'42" W76°8'36"

39

Watkins Regional Park

This campground is extremely underused, so privacy is almost guaranteed.

Much like its county neighbor, Cosca Regional Park (see page 110), Watkins Regional enjoys a reputation as a beloved oasis of recreation in the congested national capital region. It encompasses more than 850 acres and has an endless array of terrific nature programs year-round, plenty of heavily wooded trails, and a wonderful nature center. In addition, the park has a popular miniature train, miniature golf, and the simply delightful Chesapeake Carousel—more than a century old—which has been entertaining youngsters (including the author of this book, many years ago) in its current location for more than 40 years. These attractions are available during summer. Visitors will also find the Old Maryland Farm, an agricultural

educational farm; athletic fields; picnic pavilions; and a popular indoor tennis bubble. There are almost 7 miles of hiking trails, plus an equestrian trail. With all of this activity—and the park is well used—the idea of camping here might seem completely anathema. Not so fast. While the campground is primitive, it is surprisingly quiet and can offer a quick and perfectly lovely night out in the woods for the many residents who live close by. The campground is in a wooded section of the park, away from all the activity and amenities listed above.

Certainly compared to the campsites in this book out in the beautiful wilds of Western Maryland or the incomparable maritime beauty of the Eastern Shore and Atlantic Coast, Watkins simply doesn't measure up. But these (sub)urban parks with campgrounds provide a valuable resource, and a night or two here can be just the ticket for a terrific mini-vacation. (And let's be honest: If you have kids with you, you'll be grateful for the above attractions. There's plenty to do in this park to keep everyone perfectly happy for a weekend.) Best of all, the campground is incredibly underused, so privacy is almost

:: Ratings

BEAUTY: ★ ★ ★
PRIVACY: ★ ★ ★ ★
SPACIOUSNESS: ★ ★ ★
QUIET: ★ ★ ★ ★
SECURITY: ★ ★ ★ ★ ★
CLEANLINESS: ★ ★

:: Key Information

ADDRESS: Watkins Regional Park
301 Watkins Park Drive
Upper Marlboro, MD 20774

CONTACT: 301-218-6700

OPERATED BY: Maryland-National
Capital Park and Planning Commission, Prince George's County Department of Parks and Recreation

OPEN: Year-round

SITES: 34

EACH SITE: Picnic table, fire ring,
trash can

ASSIGNMENT: First come, first served

REGISTRATION: At the Watkins Tennis
Bubble on Saturday and Sunday,
9 a.m.–7 p.m., or at 301-218-6870

FACILITIES: Bathhouse and water. In
park: playgrounds, pavilions, tennis,

museum, carousel, miniature golf,
nature center

PARKING: At site

FEE: Seniors: $10/night; Prince
George's and Montgomery County
residents: $12/night; nonresidents:
$20/night

RESTRICTIONS

▓ **Pets:** Allowed on leash

▓ **Quiet Hours:** 10 p.m.–7 a.m.

▓ **Visitors:** Maximum 6 people/site.
Exceptions can be obtained for immediate families of more than 6 people.

▓ **Fires:** In fire rings

▓ **Alcohol:** Not permitted

▓ **Stay Limit:** 2 weeks within any
4-week period

▓ **Other:** Reservations must be made
within 30 days of visit. Checkout noon.

guaranteed. For example, when I visited on a weekend in August, only 5 of the 34 sites were occupied.

To get your spot, call or visit the tennis bubble and let the staff know which site you wish to reserve. If it's vacant, it's yours. The campground has one unpaved loop road with the sites staggered within and around the circle. There is relatively little to distinguish one from another. However, I would concentrate on sites 6–14. Of these, 8 and 10 seem the best; 8 has a nice little stream behind it, and both 8 and 10 are comparatively large and nicely wooded. I would avoid 4, as it has a little path through it that

connects to site 31, on the other end of the loop. Around site 14, you will begin to hear the road noise from nearby MD 193. This remains true as you continue along the sites through to number 22. Only at 23/24 does the road noise begin to die away. (Note that MD 193, while a major road, isn't a super highway, so "road noise" is a relative term.) The bathhouse sits between sites 23 and 25, so this can be either a bonus or something you want to avoid. No site in the loop is very far from the bathhouse, so my preference would be to stay on the other side of the loop, sites 8–14, as noted above. (The one exception to this might be site 29; if you

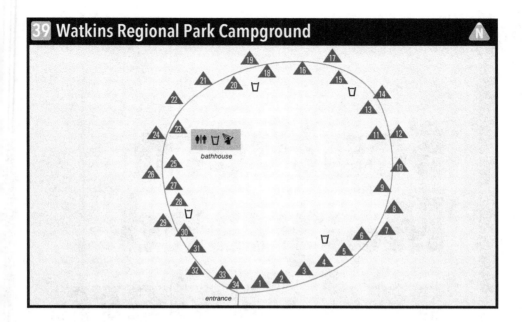

39 Watkins Regional Park Campground

bathhouse

entrance

are a large group and want space, nab this one, as it's huge compared to the rest in the campground.) As for the bathhouse itself, it isn't new, but it's kept clean and is more than serviceable. The campground itself does have some trash strewn about here and there (despite each site having a large trash can), thus the lower score for cleanliness. But it's nothing too terrible. In short, Watkins is an easy and pleasant getaway for folks in an otherwise crowded region.

:: Getting There

From I-495, take Exit 15A/MD 214 E/Central Avenue. Head east on MD 214/Central Avenue, and go 2.9 miles. Turn right onto Watkins Park Drive (MD 193). The park will be on the right.

GPS COORDINATES N38°53'14.9" W76°47'12.7"

Southern Maryland and Eastern Shore

40

Assateague Island National Seashore: Bayside Campground

The name Assateague is known all over the country as the "place with the wild horses."

Assateague Island is a barrier island, stretching 37 miles from just south of Ocean City all the way to Chincoteague in Virginia. It's very narrow in places; this allows for watching the sunrise over the Atlantic and then turning around later in the day and watching it set over Sinepuxent or Chincoteague Bay.

The name Assateague is known all over the country as the "place with the wild horses." Indeed, they're all over the island, though the Virginia (known as Chincoteague ponies) and Maryland herds are kept separate. First-time visitors to Assateague are often amazed when they spot one of the animals; by the end of the visit, they've probably fought more than one urge to shoo them away from

their campsite or off the road. The horses have certainly gotten used to humans and show no fear (I still have a vivid memory of being horrified when, as a little boy, I was in the back seat of a car when one stuck his snout in the window and held it inches from my face). The horses are stout (read: short and fat) and don't inspire images of free-riding Western plains Wildfires. Still, they are a sight. Their presence helps to make Assateague a truly special place— and certainly a must-camp destination for any Marylander. Though Marylanders do indeed make up the bulk of Assateague's campers, you'll find visitors from all over the country.

Assateague Island National Seashore is divided into two separate camping areas: Oceanside and Bayside, logically named because of their respective locations. The Oceanside has double the sites because it's more popular. Nevertheless, campers— especially repeat campers who always go for the Oceanside sites—should give the Bayside a try. Certainly, if you desire shade in the hot summer months, the Bayside sites provide much more of it than

:: Ratings

BEAUTY: ★ ★ ★ ★ ★
PRIVACY: ★ ★ ★
SPACIOUSNESS: ★ ★ ★
QUIET: ★ ★ ★
SECURITY: ★ ★ ★ ★ ★
CLEANLINESS: ★ ★ ★ ★

:: Key Information

ADDRESS: Assateague Island National Seashore, 7206 National Seashore Lane Berlin, MD 21811

CONTACT: 410-641-3030; **nps.gov/asis**

OPERATED BY: National Park Service

OPEN: Year-round

SITES: 49

EACH SITE: Picnic table, grill, fire ring

ASSIGNMENT: Reservations required mid-March–mid-November; first come, first served otherwise

REGISTRATION: Self-register at North Beach Ranger Station, call 877-444-6777, or visit **recreation.gov**

FACILITIES: Chemical toilets, cold-water showers, drinking water

PARKING: 2 vehicles maximum; parking off Bayberry Drive for walk-in sites

FEE: $30/night, plus $15 park entrance fee (good for 7 days)

RESTRICTIONS

Pets: Permitted but must be leashed and attended

Quiet Hours: 10 p.m.–6 a.m.

Visitors: 6 persons (or immediate family) maximum

Fires: Allowed on the beach below high-tide line but not at campsites

Alcohol: Not permitted

Stay Limit: Total of 28 nights/year, only 14 during reservation season

Other: Illegal to feed or approach wildlife ($500 fine); check-in noon; checkout 11 a.m.

the Oceanside ones, which offer virtually none. However, it is much more buggy on the Bayside in summer. This detriment, combined with the magnetic pull of the ocean, means that the Bayside is often the consolation for those who couldn't get an Oceanside site. However, there are some real advantages to the Bayside sites. If your reasons for coming include wildlife-viewing, birding, or canoeing/kayaking, the Bayside is the better bet. Because of the increased vegetation, the area is a birder's paradise. Plus, the Bayside has the national seashore's boat launch and can have fires in the fire pits (there are only grills at the Oceanside campsites).

The Bayside Campground has three loops: A, B, and C. Each of the three loops

has a shower and restroom. A nice feature of the Bayside Campground is the bicycle and canoe rental, at the westernmost end of the campground, past Loop C at the Bayside Picnic Area. Loop A has sites 1–24, B has 25–37, and C contains 38–49, so no one loop is terribly big. If you most desire quiet, shoot for Loop B, as generators are prohibited there. The best site in the campground is in B: site 35. It overlooks a beautiful little sandy beach. If you can't get 35, try to get one of the nearby ones (33 and 37 are good).

Because the Sinepuxent Bay wraps around the entire peninsula where the Bayside sites are located, no site is very far from the water. However, the main camp road does sit between some sites

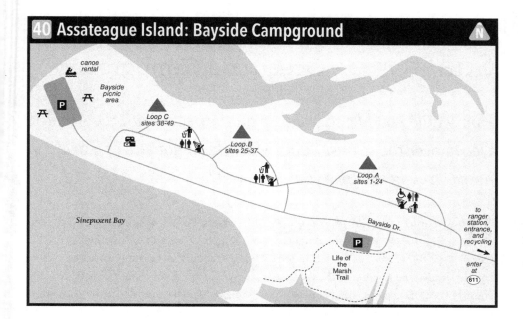

and the bay. If you want a site without that barrier, go for the sites on the western side of the three loops. Specifically, this means 14, 15, 17, 18, 20, 22, and 24 in Loop A (of these, sites 22 and 24 are closest); 33, 35, and 37 in Loop B; and 45, 46, and 48 in Loop C (though 47 and 49 aren't bad either).

:: Getting There

From the intersection of US 113 and US 50 in Berlin, head east on US 50, and go 6.1 miles. Turn right on MD 611, and travel south 8.3 miles to the park entrance. Once in the park, turn right on Stephen Decatur Memorial Road, and go 2.3 miles to Bayside Campground on the right.

GPS COORDINATES N38°12'18.3" W75°09'14.2"

41

Assateague Island National Seashore: Oceanside Campground

How would you like to wake up on the beach with the Atlantic Ocean over the closest dune, while the silhouette of a wild horse stretches across your tent wall?

How would you like to wake up on the beach with the Atlantic Ocean over the closest dune, while the silhouette of a wild horse stretches across your tent wall? Sound like paradise? It's pretty close, and it's well worth the relentless mosquitoes. It's Assateague Island National Seashore.

Oceanside campsites at Assateague Island can be tough to get. Everyone's clamoring for a spot in the sand just 100 feet from the Atlantic. (You should note, however, that the campsites are in the dunes, so the ocean won't be visible from your tent.) Even summer's heat and biting bugs aren't enough to deter the crowds. They come for the sunrises,

:: Ratings

BEAUTY: ★ ★ ★ ★ ★
PRIVACY: ★ ★ ★
SPACIOUSNESS: ★ ★ ★
QUIET: ★ ★ ★
SECURITY: ★ ★ ★ ★ ★
CLEANLINESS: ★ ★ ★ ★

sunsets, horses, swimming, fishing, crabbing, boating, and off-roading.

Though not as much of a draw, hiking is a must, but for those not used to walking along a barrier island, there are some must-know things. One of my earliest memories involves hiking out in nearby Toms Cove (on Chincoteague Island, in Virginia) during a trip to Assateague; we walked and walked, seemingly for miles, and the water barely reached up to our waists. Then, quite suddenly, it got higher and higher as we ran back, barely reaching shore before the water was over our heads. Also, so much standing water brings out mosquitoes in droves. Gnats and ticks are constant pests as well. Wind is something else people complain about. Make sure to bring sand stakes for your tent—short stakes could mean your tent gets blown away.

Nevertheless, the crowds come, and it's easy to see why. Without question, the best bets are the Oceanside walk-in sites. These are tent-only and are all within 200 feet of parking areas. It's a great setup.

:: Key Information

ADDRESS: Assateague Island National Seashore, 7206 National Seashore Lane Berlin, MD 21811

CONTACT: 410-641-3030; **nps.gov/asis**

OPERATED BY: National Park Service

OPEN: Year-round

SITES: 104

EACH SITE: Picnic table, grill, fire ring

ASSIGNMENT: Reservations required mid-March–mid-November; first come, first served otherwise

REGISTRATION: Self-register at North Beach Ranger Station, call 877-444-6777, or visit **recreation.gov**

FACILITIES: Chemical toilets, cold-water showers, drinking water

PARKING: 2 vehicles maximum; parking areas off Bayberry Drive for walk-in sites

FEE: $30/night, plus $15 park entrance fee (good for 7 days)

RESTRICTIONS:

Pets: Permitted but must be leashed and attended

Quiet Hours: 10 p.m.–6 a.m.

Visitors: 6 persons (or immediate family) maximum

Fires: Allowed on the beach below high-tide line but not at campsites

Alcohol: Not permitted

Stay Limit: Total of 28 nights/year, only 14 during reservation season

Other: Illegal to feed or approach wildlife ($500 fine); check-in noon; checkout 11 a.m.

Leave your car at the lot, and then walk to the site, right on the beach. Some privacy is lost, but this is a natural function of the topography; in most cases, sand separates you and the next tent, as opposed to a tree buffer. However, the sites are surprisingly well spaced and can even feel private. The Oceanside walk-ins number 42–104. The best of the best are sites 99–104 (more private), which lie on the eastern end of the Oceanside Area on South Ocean Beach and leave virtually nothing between you and the ocean. Also good are sites 85 and 94–98. Life of the Dunes Nature Trail sits at the end of this area, beyond the camp roads. Also, if you happen to be bringing your own horse with you (as opposed to the wild horses that make the area famous), there are two horse campsites on the eastern edge, near the mid-80s sites. These sites contain room for six people and as many horses.

Also included in the Oceanside Campground are Loop 1 (sites 1–19) and Loop 2 (sites 20–41); these loops are drive-in. The pleasant Life of the Forest Trail sits across Ocean Drive and Bayberry Drive from sites 20–24 in the drive-in section and 42–46 of the walk-in area. (There's also a Life of the Marsh nature trail, off Bayside

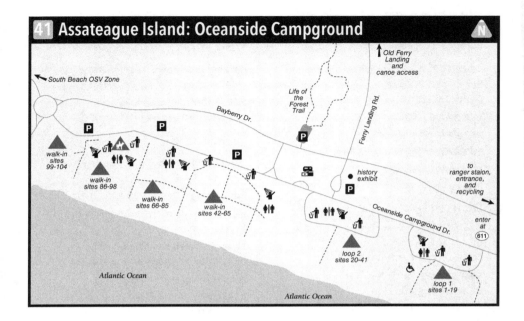

Drive, near Bayside Campground.) Six well-spaced shower-and-restroom facilities serve Oceanside Campground.

Again, getting a site in the popular months is tough enough (book as far in advance as you can), so take what's available. But if you do have your pick of spots, consider the following. While you can dive into the Atlantic anywhere you like, a lifeguard beach (North Ocean Beach) sits closest to the entrance to Loop 1; if you have young kids, this might be the wisest choice. If you want more privacy and easy access to the trails along the island heading south toward Chincoteague, go for the tent-only sites at the end of the loop, on South Ocean Beach. Last, if clamming, crabbing, and boating are more your thing, the road to Old Ferry Landing sits across from Loop 2, past the visitor center (well worth a visit itself).

:: Getting There

From the intersection of US 113 and US 50 in Berlin, head east on US 50, and go 6.1 miles. Turn right on MD 611, and travel south 8.5 miles to the park entrance. Turn right on Stephen Decatur Memorial Road, and go 2.5 miles.

GPS COORDINATES N38°12'15.2" W75°09'10.1"

42

Assateague Island National Seashore: Backcountry Sites

This unforgettable experience is well worth the work of getting here.

The backcountry campsites at Assateague Island National Seashore are not for the faint of heart; they are reached only after a decent walk or paddle and require that you haul in all your gear, even water. Those who do undertake the trip are rewarded with an unparalleled experience—a stunning (and often empty) beach where, on a clear night, accompanied by the soft lap of Atlantic waves, one can gaze into a sky full of stars unimpeded by artificial light. It's like stepping back a century, and it offers an unforgettable experience, well worth the work of getting there. You should be aware, however, that unpredictable weather conditions mean that rangers may close off the entire backcountry area.

:: Ratings

BEAUTY: ★ ★ ★ ★ ★
PRIVACY: ★ ★ ★
SPACIOUSNESS: ★ ★ ★ ★
QUIET: ★ ★ ★ ★
SECURITY: ★ ★ ★ ★
CLEANLINESS: ★ ★ ★ ★ ★

Also, you'll have to sign a waiver acknowledging that rescue personnel may not be able to come get you if something goes wrong. Last, you have to be prepared to pack everything in and out; the backcountry of the seashore demands Leave No Trace ethics.

Assateague Island National Seashore has two oceanside backcountry campsites (Little Levels and State Line). Short trails off the beach take you there; from the ranger station, it's 4 miles to Little Levels and a haul of 11 miles to State Line. (This varies if you are coming from Tom's Cove in Virginia—from the south, in other words—as opposed to the north; see below.) There are also four bayside sites (Tingles Island, Pine Tree, Green Run, and Pope Bay), which can be reached by canoe or kayak. Distances to the bayside campsites are more manageable for several reasons. First, obviously, your transport can be your water vessel, as opposed to your feet. Second, you have four to choose from instead of just two, which leads to the third reason: shorter distances.

:: Key Information

ADDRESS: Assateague Island National Seashore, 7206 National Seashore Lane Berlin, MD 21811

CONTACT: 410-641-3030; **nps.gov/asis**

OPERATED BY: National Park Service

OPEN: Year-round, but sites occasionally may be closed due to extreme weather. In spring and summer, one or both backcountry oceanside sites may be closed due to bird nesting. Bayside sites are open all year except briefly during hunting season in autumn (call 410-641-3030 for hunting dates). The NPS does not recommend camping on the bayside in summer because of high concentrations of biting insects.

SITES: 6, each holding 10-25 people

EACH SITE: Picnic tables, fire rings

ASSIGNMENT: First come, first served

REGISTRATION: At North Beach Ranger Station

FACILITIES: Chemical toilets

PARKING: All vehicles must be left at the North Beach Ranger Station for hikers and the Old Ferry Landing Parking Area or Bayside Picnic Area for paddlers.

FEE: $6/person backcountry permit plus $15 park entrance fee/vehicle (good for 7 days); obtain permits at the Assateague Island National Seashore Ranger Station

RESTRICTIONS:

▥ **Pets:** Prohibited

▥ **Quiet Hours:** 10 p.m.-6 a.m.

▥ **Visitors:** Must obtain permits

▥ **Fires:** In fire rings at bayside sites; allowed on beach below high-tide line at oceanside sites; must be extinguished with water, not sand

▥ **Alcohol:** Not permitted

▥ **Stay Limit:** Permits are good for up to 7 days and can be renewed.

▥ **Other:** No freshwater is available at any backcountry site; haul in your own water. Camp only at the site listed on your permit.

The privacy, spaciousness, and quiet ratings here are averages and depend entirely on how many people you share the space with, which will be determined mostly by time of year and distance from the headquarters. Rangers issue permits until the maximum number of accommodations for each site fills, so your privacy and space will obviously depend on the number of people filling the spaces. For individual sites, vacancy is determined by the following formula: Little Levels and State Line have no limit on the number of groups but max out at 30 and 25 people, respectively (meaning that there may be up to 25 individual campers, or one group of 25, or anything in between). Tingles Island and Pine Tree can have five groups and/or 25 people, Green Run can have three groups and/or 15 people, and Pope Bay can have two groups and/or 10 people.

Check-in times vary by site; rangers issue permits based on the distance one has to travel to get to the site. Based on sunset time, these check-in times will obviously vary over the course of the year. But the following holds steady no matter what time of year: Check-in is two hours before sunset for Tingles Island, Little Levels, and Pine Tree and four hours before sunset for Green Run, State Line, and Pope Bay. As noted above, check-in times, as well as distances to campsites and required parking areas, differ if you're coming from Virginia. Visit **assateagueisland.com** for Virginia information and distances.

Not surprisingly, State Line offers the most solitude, as relatively few people are willing to hike 13 miles with camping equipment. If you are, your rewards will be plentiful; the Atlantic is simply and unfailingly beautiful. Little Levels, because it's closer, is more popular. But even if all space gets filled, something wonderful often happens in places like this. While small campsites in forests often lead to a natural inclination to seal yourself within your space (after all, why did you choose to leave your warm and comfortable bed to sleep in the woods?), on an open beach, with fires roaring, it's almost impossible not to feel that you and your neighbors, here at the end of the earth, are in on something grand and communal. Assateague's backcountry spaces may well be the only places where you might feel better having lots of neighbors. Then again, maybe not—and if not, go for the State Line section, where your chances for lots of neighbors decrease.

It's important to note that rangers do not recommend summer camping in the bayside sites, which are havens for swarms of biting insects (mosquitoes mostly, but all those horses running around ensure some nasty horseflies too). There's one annoyance to the oceanside sites, as well, though it certainly shouldn't deter you: The beach from the ranger station to the state line is an Over Sand Vehicle zone. Expect to see permitted trucks churning up and down the beach. These can certainly shatter the harmony of an oceanside hike along the water line, but all the "traffic" is mandated to be gone by the time you bed down for the night.

While many oceanside sites offer the attraction of sleeping near the ocean, the bayside sites—aside from Pope Bay—offer forest and shade. While this is an important consideration, your destination should probably depend on how much paddling you're willing or wanting to do to get there: Tingles Island requires a paddle of 3 miles, Pine Tree is 6 miles, Green Run is 10.5 miles, and Pope Bay is a trip of 14 miles.

Tingles Island can be quick and easy, and you'll be on the edge of beautiful Tingles Narrows, studded with little islands that hum with birdsong. Pine Tree requires you to pass through Tingles Narrows before an easy take-out at the campsite. Green Run sits at the tip of Green Run Bay, a cove just beyond the Pirate Islands. Last is Pope Bay, which sits in the bay of the same name and is

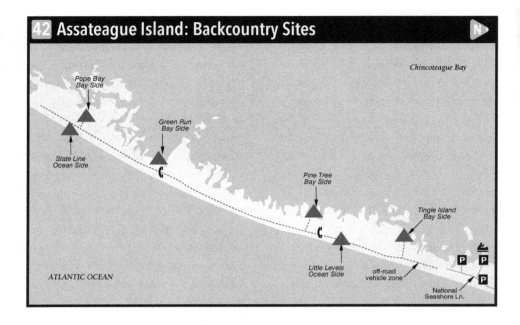

42 Assateague Island: Backcountry Sites

a wonderful kayak trip. Getting there requires weaving through lots of marshland alive with waterfowl—well worth the strenuous trip. In the case of these bayside backcountry sites, getting there can be half the fun.

:: Getting There

From the intersection of US 113 and US 50 in Berlin, head east on US 50, and go 6.1 miles. Turn right on MD 611, and travel south 8.5 miles to the park entrance. Turn right on Stephen Decatur Memorial Road, and go 2.5 miles. Park at the North Beach Campground parking if hiking in. If paddling in, go 3 miles along Stephen Decatur, and turn right on Ferry Landing Road. Refer to the text and **assateagueisland.com** for directions to sites from there.

GPS COORDINATES N38°12'15.2" W75°09'10.1"

43

Assateague State Park

National Geographic Traveler *once selected Assateague State Park as 1 of the 10 best state parks in America.*

Not to be confused with Assateague Island National Seashore, Assateague State Park is run by the Maryland Department of Natural Resources. In what's an oft-quoted boast, *National Geographic Traveler* magazine once selected Assateague State Park as 1 of the 10 best state parks in America. Assateague State Park is the only ocean park in the state parks system, hemmed in by the Atlantic on one side and Sinepuxent Bay on the other, located on Assateague Island.

Those who have been camping here for decades can remember the days when the campsites were in full view of the ocean. That is no longer the case, but it's for a very good reason: massive erosion. The dunes have been restored; while they cut off the view (there are paths between

:: Ratings

BEAUTY: ★ ★ ★ ★ ★
PRIVACY: ★ ★ ★
SPACIOUSNESS: ★ ★ ★
QUIET: ★ ★ ★
SECURITY: ★ ★ ★ ★ ★
CLEANLINESS: ★ ★ ★ ★

dunes), the restoration was essential for the fragile ecosystem the park hosts. The dunes are integral to protecting the island, just as the island is integral to protecting the mainland.

Owing to its popularity, Assateague State Park has some 350 campsites spread over 10 loops (A–J). Don't expect to have the place to yourself. Worse, in summer, you'd be willing to trade the mosquitoes for another thousand people. Still, a book on Maryland camping must include Assateague. Simply put, it's a special place. Deer and wild ponies wander the area like animals used to human contact (which, of course, they are). This can create some problems, such as when they are unwilling to leave your campsite or get out of the way of your car. There are strict policies against feeding or touching any animals.

Loop A has 22 sites and a bathhouse. Sites 10–15 are closest to the ocean. Note, however, that "closest to the ocean" means some 40 yards or so—nothing too terrible, but this is true of all the camp loops. Sites 1, 2, 21, and 22 are nearest the main camp road, Ocean Drive. All sites are a decent size, but if you require room, the biggest in Loop A are 2 and 22, both

:: Key Information

ADDRESS: Assateague State Park
6915 Stephen Decatur Highway
Berlin, MD 21811

CONTACT: 410-641-2120;
dnr2.maryland.gov

OPERATED BY: Maryland Department of Natural Resources

OPEN: Late April–late October

SITES: 350

EACH SITE: Fire ring, picnic table

ASSIGNMENT: Reservations recommended

REGISTRATION: 888-432-CAMP (2267) or **reservations.dnr.state.md.us**

FACILITIES: Boat launch, camp store, dump station, vending, nature center

PARKING: In paved spots at each site (3 units maximum)

FEE: $27.49 plus service charge/night; $38.49 plus service charge/night electric; additional day-use service charge during high season: $4–$6

RESTRICTIONS

- **Pets:** Allowed in Loop J, Loop I sites 37-51, and Loop H
- **Quiet Hours:** 11 p.m.–7 a.m.
- **Visitors:** Register vehicle and name at ranger station, 6 people maximum
- **Fires:** In fire rings only; not allowed on beach
- **Alcohol:** Permitted only inside cabins and at shelters with valid permit, as applicable
- **Stay Limit:** None
- **Other:** Check-in 2 p.m.; checkout 11 a.m.

of which sit on the internal loop immediately after entering from Ocean Drive.

Loop B has 24 sites. Sites 9–15 are closest to the ocean, and 1, 2, 23, and 24 are nearest Ocean Drive. B shares a bathhouse with Loop C. The two largest sites in B are 22 and 12.

Loop C has 24 sites. Sites 12 and 13 are closest to the ocean, and 1, 2, 23, and 24 are nearest Ocean Drive. The largest sites are 13 and 20. Site 13 also sits on the northeastern corner of the loop road, nearest the ocean, so it's a nice spot.

Loop D has 28 sites, a bathhouse, and sits adjacent to the nature center.

Sites 14–17 are closest to the beach, and 1, 2, 27, and 28 are nearest Ocean Drive. Sites 13–17 are smaller than the rest, which look pretty uniform in size.

Loops E–G have sites that are generally larger than those found in A–D. Loop E contains a bathhouse (sites 14–18 are closest to the ocean, and 1, 2, 3, and 30 are nearest Ocean Drive); Loop F has a bathhouse and 30 sites. Sites 4, 6, 8, and 10 are wheelchair accessible (sites 15–19 are closest to the ocean, and 1 and 2 are near Ocean Drive). Note that 2016 renovations to bathhouses 6–9 will affect loops G, H, I, and J (see individual notes following).

Loop G will be unavailable for reservations during renovations; otherwise, it has 30 sites (sites 14–17 are closest to the ocean, and 1, 2, and 30 are nearest Ocean Drive; additionally, sites 7–11 sit near the bathhouse and a dumping station). Loop H has 39 sites, all of them electric, so if tent camping, skip Loop H; if you do wind up here, however, note that portable bathrooms will be available during the bathhouse renovations. Loop I has two bathhouses and an astounding, tightly packed 110 sites. The sites aren't much smaller than those in E–G, but there are just so many folks with whom you have to share the loop. That said, many of those sites will be unavailable during the bathhouse renovations, specifically sites 1–35 and 73–110.

In my opinion, the best option is Loop J, the southernmost loop. No one else will be driving past your campsite, as J is the end and contains only 13 sites,

as well as a bathhouse (though this will be replaced by portable toilets during renovation. Of course, all campers are allowed to use bathhouses 1–5 in Loops A–F). Sites 11, 12, and 13 may be the best in the entire park because they sit closest to the ocean. The sites here are a little smaller than elsewhere in the park, but there's certainly room enough, and what you give up in space is worth it.

With so many spots, it's difficult to recommend many specific ones. It might be best to consult the campground map and make your decision based on your particular wants and needs, such as proximity to bathhouses or ocean. There is one last consideration to help guide you. For the sandiest spots, which many people find attractive because they give the best sense of the ocean, head to Loop A. If you prefer more vegetation, which provides the advantage of potential shade, go for Loop E or F.

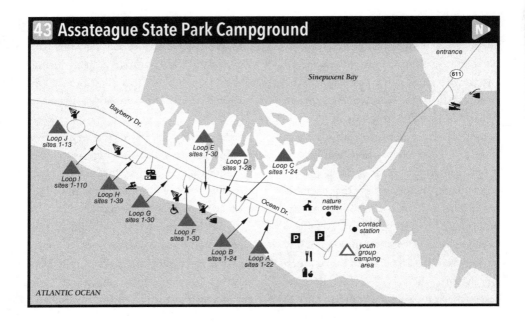

:: Getting There

From the intersection of US 113 and US 50 in Berlin, head east on US 50, and go 6.1 miles. Turn right on MD 611, and travel south 8.5 miles to the park entrance. Turn right, and the campground is on the left.

GPS COORDINATES N38°14'02.5" W75°08'17.5"

44

Janes Island State Park

Spend some time in picture-perfect tidewater Maryland.

Note: **Construction will be** ongoing at Janes Island through at least winter 2016 and includes the renovation of bathhouse B and the addition of full-service cabins. In 2015 renovations to the nature center and park store were completed. Call the park before visiting in case construction completion is delayed and to see how construction noise and activity might impact camping.

Janes Island State Park, at 3,147 acres, is thought of in two parts: the developed section and the outlying, rugged area accessible only by boat. And in between? Picture-perfect tidewater Maryland. As an added bonus, thousands of migrating waterfowl that stop over at nearby Blackwater National Wildlife Refuge can be easily spotted in and around Janes Island. It is, in a word, beautiful.

America's history is inextricably linked with Maryland's, and that may be truer of the area around Janes Island than anywhere else. Settled in 1658 by English colonists, it was first explored by John Smith the year after Jamestown was settled. Smith, no doubt, came upon the original inhabitants, Annemessex American Indians. To this day, Annemessex artifacts can be found on nearby Smith Island. From nearby Crisfield, the "end of the land," you can get a ferry to Smith Island, the no-stoplight place where, purportedly, the locals speak the New World's closest thing to British English. The local twang doesn't sound very British to me, but many of the island's residents can trace their lineage to those first English settlers.

Janes Island has been designated part of the Chesapeake Bay Gateway, a series of parks, wildlife refuges, museums, ships, historic communities, and trails—"special places where you can experience the authentic Chesapeake." Janes Island is also part of the Beach to Bay Indian Trail, stretching 55 miles from the Atlantic to the Bay, roughly following American Indian trails.

This is a water park, dominated by Tangier Sound to the west and the Big Annemessex River to the north. Accordingly, Janes Island offers six water trails: Red, Brown, Yellow, Green, Black, and Blue. Each offers unique access to area

:: Ratings

BEAUTY: ★ ★ ★ ★ ★
PRIVACY: ★ ★ ★ ★
SPACIOUSNESS: ★ ★ ★
QUIET: ★ ★ ★ ★
SECURITY: ★ ★ ★ ★ ★
CLEANLINESS: ★ ★ ★ ★

:: Key Information

ADDRESS: Janes Island State Park
26280 Alfred J. Lawson Drive
Crisfield, MD 21817

CONTACT: 410-968-1565;
dnr2.maryland.gov

OPERATED BY: Maryland Department
of Natural Resources

OPEN: Late March–December

SITES: 107

EACH SITE: Picnic table, fire ring,
lantern post

ASSIGNMENT: Reservations
recommended

REGISTRATION: 888-432-CAMP
(2267) or reservations.dnr.state.md.us

FACILITIES: Boat launch and rental,
camp store, conference center, dump
station, playground, visitor center

PARKING: At designated spots

FEE: $21.49 plus service charge/night;
$27.49 plus service charge/night elec-
tric; boat launch $7/vehicle; boat launch
for out-of-state residents $9/vehicle

RESTRICTIONS

▪ **Pets:** Allowed in loops A and B

▪ **Quiet Hours:** 11 p.m.–7 a.m.

▪ **Visitors:** Must register if staying overnight; otherwise, must leave by 11 p.m.

▪ **Fires:** No open fires

▪ **Alcohol:** Permitted only inside
cabins and at shelters with valid
permit, as applicable

▪ **Stay Limit:** None

▪ **Other:** Mosquitoes are serious business at Janes Island. Camping here
without defense can ruin your stay. Try
the insect repellent from Burt's Bees.

waterways; the Blue Trail, for instance, takes in Ward Creek, the Daugherty Creek Canal, and the Little Annemessex River. The Black, Blue, Red, and Yellow Trails all wind through the creeks and marshland within the island. The Green and Brown Trails head all the way out to Tangier Sound and are for experienced paddlers. With all these options, you'll be satisfied no matter what your skill level. Three primitive backcountry campsites are available along the water trails, each with tent platforms and boat landings: one on the north side, one on the south side, and one in the middle of the island. Each is accessible only by canoe or kayak and requires you to pack out everything. One word of

warning if roughing it appeals to you: The mosquitoes are worse here than in the campground (if that can be believed). But it may be worth braving the bugs; these are beautiful sites and rather private. To camp here, you must obtain a permit from the park headquarters.

You enter the park on Alfred J. Lawson Drive and head straight toward Daugherty Creek Canal, which gives access to the water trails. Loop A is the closest to all the action: the marina, boat launch, bathhouse, trailer storage, etc. No matter where you stay in the campground, you'll come this way when it's time to launch. Loop A contains sites 41–66, and all allow pets. Sites 47–51 are the most pleasant if

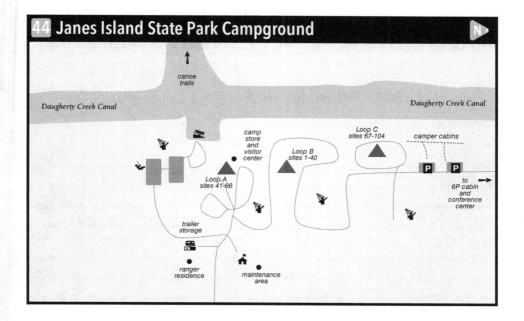

44 Janes Island State Park Campground

canoe trails

Daugherty Creek Canal

Daugherty Creek Canal

camp store and visitor center

Loop A
sites 41-66

Loop B
sites 1-40

Loop C
sites 67-104

camper cabins

P P

to
6P cabin
and
conference
center

trailer
storage

ranger
residence

maintenance
area

you're looking for space from your neighbors; however, they are all electric (none of the others in Loop A are).

Relatively small Loop B contains sites 1–40 and is tucked up toward the canal from the roads leading to and from Loops A and C. This is Janes Island's electric loop. Pets are allowed in sites 1–13 and 23–40, and sites 13–16 are wheelchair accessible.

Loop C (sites 67–104) contains the park's best sites, but no pets are allowed in this loop. It is almost entirely nonelectric, with the exception of sites 70–73, which sit by themselves. Because of their nonelectric status and proximity to the water, the best of the best are sites 74–79, which sit on the outside loop near Daugherty Creek Canal. My favorite site in the park, however, is 81, which also sits by the water but does not have the loop road in between, making it your best bet for privacy.

:: Getting There

From the intersection of US 50 and US 13 north of Salisbury, head southeast on US 50, and go 3.5 miles. Continue on US 13 S, and go 20.2 miles. Turn right on MD 413 S, and go 11.3 miles. Turn right on Plantation Road (which becomes Jacksonville Road). After 1.5 miles, take a right on Alfred Lawson Drive and reach the park in 0.5 mile.

GPS COORDINATES   N38°0'59" W75°51'27"

45

Martinak State Park

Special programs make Martinak a family-friendly camping experience.

On the site of a former Indian village, Martinak State Park is small at only 107 acres, but that's partly because it's hemmed in by so much water. Bordered by the Choptank River (the Chesapeake's largest Eastern Shore tributary) and Watts Creek, Martinak is understandably popular as a fishing and boating haven. Bass, catfish, perch, and sunfish are the popular catches in and around the park (you must have a Chesapeake Bay Sportfishing License). Hardwood and pine forests surround both waterways, providing great hiking and birding. A birding camp in July and a bass-fishing camp in August will teach you how to increase your chances in both.

Other special programs help make Martinak family friendly. A youth fishing derby, a junior ranger program, and Summer Park Pals for 4- to 6-year-olds are just some of Martinak State Park's special events. Summer concerts and country auctions also pull people from all over the Eastern Shore. While the crowds these events attract might turn some people off, Martinak always feels like a friendly and pleasant place to be. In fact, most campers you'll meet at Martinak are folks who return year after year, giving the place a fraternal feel.

In the last decade or so, Martinak has seen an upgrade in many of its facilities, as well as the addition of new trails and walkways. Part of this largesse comes from the spoils of Martinak's status as a Chesapeake Bay Gateway in a system coordinated by the National Park Service that designates Chesapeake watershed properties as worthy of protection and educational outreach. Improvements to Martinak's nature center, for example, come in part from the Gateways Network. Now, a library, aquarium, and live and stuffed animals are just part of what's to see in the nature center.

Two camping loops (A and B) serve Martinak. Loop A has sites 34–60 (plus

:: Ratings

BEAUTY: ★ ★ ★ ★
PRIVACY: ★ ★ ★ ★
SPACIOUSNESS: ★ ★ ★
QUIET: ★ ★ ★ ★
SECURITY: ★ ★ ★ ★ ★
CLEANLINESS: ★ ★ ★ ★

:: Key Information

ADDRESS: Martinak State Park, 137 Deep Shore Road, Denton, MD 21629

CONTACT: 410-820-1668; **dnr2.maryland.gov**

OPERATED BY: Maryland Department of Natural Resources

OPEN: Late March–December

SITES: 63

EACH SITE: Camping pad, picnic table, fire ring

ASSIGNMENT: Reservations recommended for holiday weekends

REGISTRATION: 888-432-CAMP (2267) or **reservations.dnr.state.md.us**

FACILITIES: Bathhouse, dump station, boat launch, playground, shelters, nature center

PARKING: In designated spots

FEE: $18.49 plus service charge/night; $24.49 plus service charge/night electric

RESTRICTIONS

▓ **Pets:** Allowed on leash

▓ **Quiet Hours:** 11 p.m.–7 a.m.

▓ **Visitors:** Register at camp entrance.

▓ **Fires:** In fire rings

▓ **Alcohol:** Permitted only inside cabins and at shelters with valid permit, as applicable

▓ **Stay Limit:** 2 weeks

four camper cabins, one of which is wheelchair accessible, as are tent sites 37, 38, 51, and 52), reservable for either tents or RVs, so who you get as a neighbor is something of a crapshoot. That said, electrical hookups are only in Loop B, so while there may be RVs if you choose Loop A, you will minimize noise. All sites sit on the outer loop; aside from the four camper cabins across from sites 47–52, there is no other camping inside the loop. Sites on the southern end of the loop (37–42) generally offer the most space between you and your neighbors. I prefer these sites, plus 43–45, for reasons of space and site depth. A hiking trail, which begins and terminates at Deep Shore Road, completely encircles the camp loop. It's easy to access the trail from anywhere in the loop.

Loop B (sites 1–27) has virtually the same setup as A, with playground equipment and a bathhouse in the middle of the loop. Of course, you will find electrical hookups in Loop B. The only other significant difference is your choice of three tent-only sites (T-1, T-2, and T-3), but they are nearest the entrance road as well as the dumpster down the street. Again, go for Loop A to avoid humming RVs; however, if you do camp in Loop B, sites 17–21 offer the best chance for some solitude. Loop B also has four wheelchair-accessible sites: 2–5. If proximity to the water (in this case, Watts Creek) is of primary interest to you, try for sites on the southern edge of

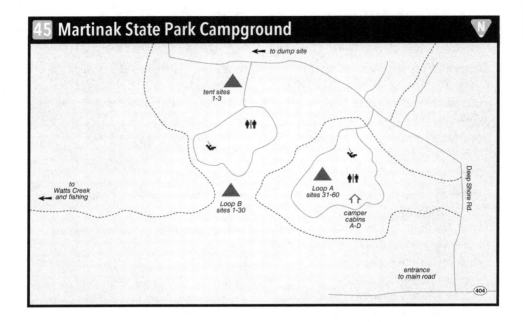

45 Martinak State Park Campground

to dump site

tent sites
1-3

to
Watts Creek
and fishing

Loop B
sites 1-30

Loop A
sites 31-60

camper
cabins
A-D

Deep Shore Rd.

entrance
to main road

404

Loop B (7–12), but, again, keep in mind that these are electric sites. Like Tuckahoe State Park (see page 177), which is administered by the same central office, the sites at Martinak are pretty uniform. They are all in nicely treed areas and have a good amount of space between them. Much thoughtfulness went into creating these sites, so all should provide a pleasant experience.

:: Getting There

From Annapolis, head east on US 50/US 301 approximately 20 miles, and take the US 50 E exit toward Ocean City. Continue on US 50 another 6.7 miles, and turn left on MD 404. In 16.1 miles turn right on Deep Shore Road. The park entrance is 0.5 mile ahead to the left.

GPS COORDINATES N38°51'45" W75°50'23"

46

Pocomoke River State Park:
Milburn Landing Area

Most Marylanders would be surprised to learn that 12 species of orchid grow in their state—and they can all be found here.

Pocomoke River State Park has two developed areas: Milburn Landing and Shad Landing. Both sit on the Pocomoke River, on opposite sides of the Pocomoke Cypress Swamp. The entire area is rather glorious, a nature-lover's paradise. Water access shouldn't necessarily be the thing that determines which of the two areas is your destination. In fact, you can paddle from one to the other (though established water trails are more abundant at Shad Landing, so Shad is arguably the better spot if your primary interest is boating). But if it's hiking you're after, Milburn allows slightly quicker access to almost 15,000 acres of wooded forest. The park's signature feature is the cypress swamps filled with the dark water of the Pocomoke

River (*Pocomoke* means "black water" in Algonquin). The Nature Conservancy owns the adjacent Nassawango Creek Preserve, which runs 9,300 acres and hosts, among other must-see wildlife, some 20 species of neotropical migratory birds.

Well-marked canoe trails are easy to follow as they wind through the swamp and tributary rivers and streams. The park is set up mostly for boaters, for good reason. Canoeing through the 30-mile Pocomoke River Swamp is a primordial experience, one that most people associate with more southern locales. In fact, Pocomoke's swamp is the northernmost example of southern cypress swamps still surviving. Most Marylanders would be surprised to learn that 12 species of orchid grow in their state—and they can all be found here. It is thought also that the swamp provided a safe haven for runaway slaves during the Civil War, as well as pirates and bootleggers. If fishing is your thing, the park's waters boast more than 50 fish species.

Those wishing for great hiking shouldn't turn away from Pocomoke.

:: Ratings

BEAUTY: ★ ★ ★ ★ ★
PRIVACY: ★ ★ ★ ★
SPACIOUSNESS: ★ ★ ★
QUIET: ★ ★ ★ ★
SECURITY: ★ ★ ★ ★ ★
CLEANLINESS: ★ ★ ★ ★ ★

:: Key Information

ADDRESS: Pocomoke River State Park
3036 Nassawango Road
Pocomoke City, MD 21851

CONTACT: 410-632-2566;
dnr2.maryland.gov

OPERATED BY: Maryland Department
of Natural Resources

OPEN: Early April–early December

SITES: 36 (including 4 mini-cabins)

EACH SITE: Picnic table, fire ring

ASSIGNMENT: Self-register at Camper
Registration Office

REGISTRATION: 888-432-CAMP
(2267), at **reservations.dnr.state
.md.us,** or on-site

FACILITIES: Bathhouse, boat launch,
dump station

PARKING: In designated spots

FEE: $18.49 plus service charge/night;
$24.49 plus service charge/night
electric

RESTRICTIONS

■ **Pets:** Permitted

■ **Quiet Hours:** 11 p.m.–7 a.m.

■ **Visitors:** Must register at registration
station; maximum 6 people/site

■ **Fires:** In fire rings

■ **Alcohol:** Permitted only inside
cabins and at shelters with valid
permit, as applicable

■ **Stay Limit:** 2 weeks; can return after
1 week away

■ **Other:** Checkout 3 p.m.

Many acres of upland forest, full of loblolly pines and spring wildflowers, offer
much to the trekker. On a waterside hike
here, I saw loads of river otters, a great
sight coming right on the heels of watching wheeling herons and eagles.

The Milburn Landing Area is much
smaller than the Shad Landing Area, with
36 sites total. It's also a bit cheaper than
Shad, but the difference is minimal, so
don't let that determine where you stay.
Better determinants include number of
facilities (Shad has much more infrastructure) and number of people (Shad
has many more of those too). In short,
if you desire more of a roughing-it feel
without the threat of large crowds, Milburn should be your choice. If you want

winter camping, which also guarantees
small numbers of people, head to Shad,
as Milburn closes by mid-December. If
you need more facilities, especially if you
have kids with you, Shad is probably the
better choice.

Ecologically, there's not much difference between the two; both offer all the
natural attractions provided by the river,
forest, streams, and swamp. And it's only
a 20-minute drive between the two sites
anyway.

Coming in off the Main Road and
passing both the boat launch and the
Camper Registration Office, you'll head
around the dump station and the road
to the state forest before coming to the
campground. Sites 1–15 sit huddled along

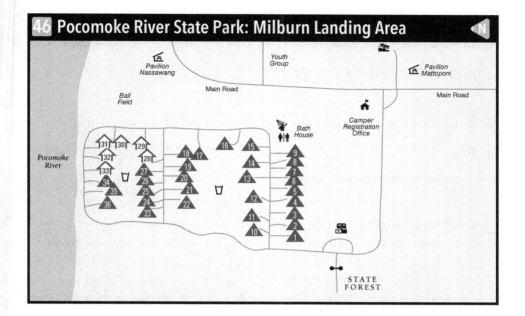

46 Pocomoke River State Park: Milburn Landing Area

the first camp road, before coming to the well-spaced and more isolated sites 16 and 17. Sites 18–27 are next, located diagonally across from one another along the camp road (sites 28–33 are cabins). Sites 34, 35, and 36 are closest to the river. Once-persistent drainage problems in this area have been addressed, so these are nice spots. Sites 1–22 provide more shade. Note, however, that most sites at Milburn are electric; these include 10–15 and 17–36. As mentioned, 16 is a nice site, but it is sandwiched between electric sites. To get as far away from potential plug-in RVs, you'll want to concentrate on sites 1–9 (the higher the number, the closer to the bathhouse; the lower the number, the closer to the entrance road).

:: Getting There

From the intersection of US 50 and US 13 north of Salisbury, head southeast on US 50, and go 3.5 miles. Continue on US 13 S, and go 28.4 miles. Turn left on MD 364, and travel 6 miles to a right into the park. In 0.5 mile turn right on River Road, and continue 1.5 miles to the campground.

GPS COORDINATES N38°07'19.6" W75°29'44"

47

Pocomoke River State Park:
Shad Landing Area

The water trail from Shad Landing to Porter's Crossing heads upriver on the Pocomoke and past Snow Hill to a remote area where civilization melts away.

Note: **Planned renovation** projects at Shad Landing, which include a new boathouse, additions to the pool, and new cabins, will be ongoing through 2016. Contact the park office to see which campsites, if any, will be affected.

Shad Landing is by far the busier of Pocomoke State Park's two developed areas. It also offers much more in the way of facilities. However, it somehow manages to remain relatively laid-back. I think it's the splendor of the area that makes people slow down and take stock.

Aside from the multitude of facilities and the abundance of campsites, two water trails distinguish Shad Landing from the smaller Milburn Landing. Because Shad Landing's campground is bordered both by the Pocomoke River and Corkers Creek, the Corkers Creek Blackwater Canoe Trail, taking in the best of the cypress swamp, is easy to access. But the granddaddy water trail is the one from Shad Landing to Porter's Crossing. This 11-mile water trail is not for the novice. It heads upriver on the Pocomoke and past Snow Hill to a remote area where civilization melts away. Of course, it's possible to access these trails from Milburn, but the additional 4.5-mile trip required to get to Shad makes the trip to Porter's Landing prohibitive for novices.

The Shad Landing area has six loops: Fox Den (A), Deer Run (B), Robin's Nest (D), Blue Heron (E), Water's Edge (F), and Acorn Trail (G), plus a youth camping area. Acorn Trail is the northernmost loop and has 30 sites, all electric, so if you're in a tent, you'd do best to avoid it. It's also closest to the busy boat launch. If you do wind up here, however, and wish for space, the largest sites in the loop are 9–12 and 20–25. Also note that pets are allowed in this loop.

:: Ratings

BEAUTY: ★ ★ ★ ★ ★
PRIVACY: ★ ★ ★ ★
SPACIOUSNESS: ★ ★ ★
QUIET: ★ ★ ★ ★
SECURITY: ★ ★ ★ ★ ★
CLEANLINESS: ★ ★ ★ ★ ★

:: Key Information

ADDRESS: Pocomoke River State Park
3461 Worcester Highway
Snow Hill, MD 21863

CONTACT: 410-632-2566;
dnr2.maryland.gov

OPERATED BY: Maryland Department of Natural Resources

OPEN: Early April–early December; Robin's Nest and Water's Edge Loops open all year for primitive camping

SITES: 175 (8 cabins)

EACH SITE: Picnic table, fire ring

ASSIGNMENT: Reservations recommended

REGISTRATION: 888-432-2267 or
reservations.dnr.state.md.us

FACILITIES: Boat launch and rental, camp store, dump station, concessions, electrical hookups, picnic areas and shelters, playgrounds, picnic shelters, swimming pool, visitor center

PARKING: In designated spots

FEE: $21.49 plus service charge/night; $27.49 plus service charge/night electric

RESTRICTIONS

- **Pets:** Allowed in Acorn Loop
- **Quiet Hours:** 11 p.m.–7 a.m.
- **Visitors:** Must register at registration station; maximum 6 people/site
- **Fires:** In fire rings
- **Alcohol:** Permitted only inside cabins and at shelters with valid permit, as applicable
- **Stay Limit:** 2 weeks; can return after 1 week away
- **Other:** Checkout 3 p.m.

Water's Edge isn't a misnomer—it sits closest to the Pocomoke and is thus among the first to fill up. It also has 30 sites (61–90). The boardwalk separates the river from sites 87 and 88. It too can get quite busy, so being so near the water might not be as desirable as you might assume. There's a marina parking lot near sites 88 and 85. Sites nearest the water are also among the smallest in the loop. The larger sites are 68–71. My recommendation is to try for site 86, which has nothing between it and the water and is sufficiently far away from the boardwalk and marina. Also nice in terms of relative privacy are sites 89 and 90.

Fox Den also has 30 sites running in a loop (31–60), with a bathhouse in the middle. Many people try to avoid sites 40 and 41 on the south end of the loop and 51–54 on the north end because a power line cut runs between them. However, people often fail to consider the nighttime view afforded by clearings. I actually like sites 52 and 53, as they sit away from the rest of the loop. The largest sites in this loop are 33, 37, 39–41, 43, and 56.

Deer Run (91–120), the next loop south of Fox Den, has 30 electric sites; avoid it if you're in a tent. If you do wind up here and space is what you are after, go for sites 101, 102, 104, 111, 112, 115, or 117.

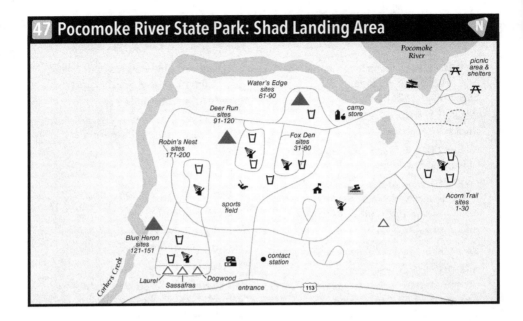

47 Pocomoke River State Park: Shad Landing Area

Robin's Nest (171–200) is a hub of activity and can get busy, with nearby ball fields and playgrounds. Additionally, the loop contains eight cabins, which can throw light and noise. However, Robin's Nest offers Shad Landing's only wheelchair-accessible camping (sites 183, 185, 195, and 200).

Blue Heron Loop (121–151) has no developed pads and is more appropriate for tent camping. A park ranger confirmed this and suggested that the best loops for tent campers are Blue Heron and Water's Edge. Another bonus of the Blue Heron Loop is that its southern edge sits close to Corkers Creek. Sites 124, 129, 135, 141, and 151 are near the water. Blue Heron also contains three family group camping sites: Laurel, Sassafras, and Dogwood.

:: Getting There

From the intersection of US 50 and US 13 north of Salisbury, head southeast on US 50, and go 3.5 miles. Continue on US 13 S, and go 3 miles to the exit for Snow Hill Road (MD 12). Turn left, and follow MD 12 for 15.2 miles. Turn right on Market Street (Business US 113), and go 3 miles. Turn right on US 113, and Shad Landing is 1.2 miles ahead on the right.

GPS COORDINATES N38°7'46" W75°26'27"

48

Point Lookout State Park

Between the camping, the swimming, the scenery, and the history, you can keep yourself joyfully occupied for days.

Point Lookout is all about the water. The entire park and campgrounds are surrounded: Lake Conoy and Point Lookout Creek split the peninsula, while the Potomac River and Chesapeake Bay meet at the southern edge. It's an exceedingly beautiful spot, though its history tells a darker tale. A Civil War prison camp on the site once housed more than 50,000 Confederate troops. Now, the place couldn't be more peaceful.

If you want hiking, you may be disappointed. The Periwinkle Point Trail (less than a mile in length) is the park's only land trail (though you can connect the park's paved roads for a hike of about 5 miles). The abundance of water and tidal action makes land trails superfluous. But if you've brought the kayak or canoe, this place is paradise. (If you didn't bring your own vessel, the camp store provides rentals on a first-come, first-serve basis.)

:: Ratings

BEAUTY: ★ ★ ★ ★ ★
PRIVACY: ★ ★ ★
SPACIOUSNESS: ★ ★ ★
QUIET: ★ ★ ★
SECURITY: ★ ★ ★ ★ ★
CLEANLINESS: ★ ★ ★ ★

Three distinct water trails lead you in and around the park: Green Points (1.7 miles) along the Lake Conoy shoreline, Heron Alley Trail (3.4 miles) through Point Lookout Creek, and Lighthouse Trail (3 miles) through tough wind-whipped open water over and around Civil War sites. Each trail can be taken as a day's highlight, or they can be combined.

If you don't have a water vessel, you need not avoid Point Lookout altogether. Between the camping, the swimming, the scenery, and the history, you can keep yourself joyfully occupied for days. There are six camp loops, hemmed in by Lake Conoy, Point Lookout Creek, and Tanner's Creek. Most of the recreational activities and infrastructure at the park are congregated toward the south of the campground, near the confluence of the Potomac and the Chesapeake. Contact stations, MD 5, and dumping and electrical hookup stations for RVs are all near the campground. Nevertheless, the sites are fairly well spaced and large, and some are very wooded. Despite the nearby activity, the place manages to feel relaxed and roomy.

The Tulip Loop (F, sites 59–83) is the northernmost and sits not too far from the

:: Key Information

ADDRESS: Point Lookout State Park
11175 Point Lookout Road
Scotland, MD 20687

CONTACT: 301-872-5688;
dnr2.maryland.gov

OPERATED BY: Maryland Department
of Natural Resources

OPEN: Late March–early November;
off-season camping available with
reduced services

SITES: 143

EACH SITE: Picnic table, fire ring

ASSIGNMENT: At camp office or park
headquarters during open hours;
self-registration otherwise

REGISTRATION: 888-432-CAMP
(2267), **reservations.dnr.state.md.us,**
or at ranger station

FACILITIES: Boat launch and rental,
camp store, bathhouses, dump station

PARKING: Each site has space for 2-3
vehicles; overflow parking available

FEE: $21.49 plus service charge/night;
$33.49 plus service charge/night electric; $38.49 plus service charge/night
water, sewer, and electric; $53.49 plus
service charge/night double sites
accommodating 12 guests; additional
day-use service charge during high
season: $3–$7, $10/vehicle; out-of-
state residents add $2

RESTRICTIONS

■ **Pets:** Leashed pets allowed in
Malone Circle, Green's Point Loop,
Tulip Loop, Hoffman's Loop

■ **Quiet Hours:** 11 p.m.–7 a.m.

■ **Visitors:** Must leave campground by
10 p.m.

■ **Fires:** In fire ring or grill

■ **Alcohol:** Permitted only inside
cabins and at shelters with valid
permit, as applicable

■ **Stay Limit:** 2 weeks; can return after
1 week away

■ **Other:** Maximum 6 people (except
sites 107 and 128, which allow 12
people); check-in and checkout 3 p.m.

road, especially sites 76–80. That said, it's heavily forested and many sites can feel quite remote when the sun goes down. However, this loop provides full electrical hookups at all sites, so it's generally best to avoid this area. If you do wind up here, sites 82, 83, and those on the western side of the Tulip Loop's entrance lane are preferable. Pets are allowed in Tulip.

The Malone Loop (E) and Green's Point Loop (B) also allow leashed pets. Green's Point (85–112) sits nearest Lake Conoy, which makes it the park's most popular loop, astride the small youth camping site (Conoy Loop [C], with six cabins). However, Green's also has full hookups, so it's probably best avoided. If you do find yourself here, sites 100–105 sit nearest the pier and have the best water access. Additionally, two wheelchair-accessible sites, 92 and 106, are available. The Malone Loop (31–57) does *not* have electrical hookups. Sites on the outer edge (44–52) offer easy access to Point Lookout's one nature trail, which is short but pleasant. Site 34 is wheelchair accessible.

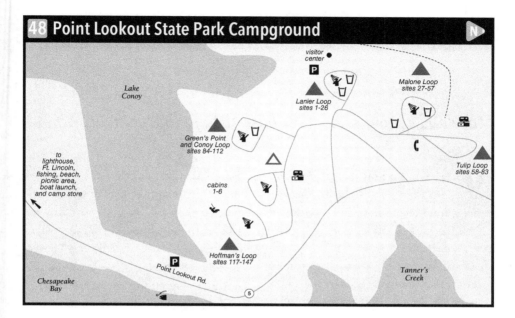

48 Point Lookout State Park Campground

Lanier Loop (D) contains 26 sites (1–26); the southwestern ones abut overflow parking and are also near the visitor center. Sites 3–15 offer the most privacy. Of these, 6 and 10 are tent-only. Another tent-only site (24) is also in Lanier Loop, and these complete Point Lookout's tent-only sites.

The final loop, Hoffman's (A, 117–146), has a few electrical sites, but they are congregated near the entrance road, on the outside of the loop (117, 119, 122, and 124). Heading to the other side of the loop, to the 130s and 140s, will keep you away from the electrical sites.

Point Lookout has a lot of campsites in a relatively small space, but this doesn't mean you won't have a pleasant experience. Again, if you've brought the boat, and especially if it's off-season, the beauty of the area and the wonderful water trails never fail to impress and inspire.

:: Getting There

From central and northern Maryland: Take I-97 to Exit 7. Continue straight on MD 3, which turns into US 301, and go 18 miles. Turn right on MD 4 S in Upper Marlboro. In 46 miles, 3 miles after crossing the Solomons Island Bridge, turn left on MD 235 S. In 16.5 miles, turn left on MD 5 S, and travel 4.7 miles to the park.

From southern Maryland and/or the D.C. area: Take I-495 to Exit 11A, and head south on MD 4. In 53.4 miles, turn left on MD 235 S, and follow the above directions.

GPS COORDINATES N38°3'30" W76°19'54"

49

Smallwood State Park

Smallwood looms large in its year-round status as Maryland's premier host for bass-fishing tournaments.

Note: **Smallwood State Park's** campground sustained heavy damage from severe storms in June 2015. Check the park's status before going in 2016 and beyond.

Smallwood State Park takes its name from its prominent early resident, Revolutionary War General William Smallwood, later Maryland's fourth governor. His house, Smallwood's Retreat (circa 1760), sits on park property and can be visited on Sundays May–September. Tours are conducted by costumed docents.

Smallwood State Park is a relatively small park at 630 acres. However, it looms large in its year-round status as Maryland's premier host for bass-fishing tournaments. Record fish are frequently pulled from the Potomac at Smallwood

State Park. Even if you're not interested in a tournament, the fishing here is sublime—and pervasive. You can fish for bass, carp, catfish, hardhead, and perch; a Chesapeake Bay Sportfishing License is required. Hiking trails are minimal, however—the entire trail system is barely 2 miles—but they do include some nice bird-watching opportunities, as well as lovely water views.

Along with its history and fishing, another Smallwood attraction is its proximity to Mattawoman Creek, a tributary of the Potomac River. The creek is duly popular with boaters and anglers using Sweden Point Marina—expect large boats, towing trucks, and RVs. In fact, all of Smallwood's 15 sites are electric. However, don't let this turn you away from this wonderful diminutive campground. With six launch slips, it's easy to squirm your way in if you have a smaller vessel. Because the campsite is small, it's never crowded (even at capacity), and the vast majority of visitors to Smallwood are day-users. Plus, it's a beautiful spot well worth a visit and not far from D.C.'s eastern suburbs.

:: Ratings

BEAUTY: ★ ★ ★ ★
PRIVACY: ★ ★ ★
SPACIOUSNESS: ★ ★ ★ ★
QUIET: ★ ★ ★ ★
SECURITY: ★ ★ ★ ★ ★
CLEANLINESS: ★ ★ ★ ★

:: Key Information

ADDRESS: Smallwood State Park
2750 Sweden Point Road
Marbury, MD 20658

CONTACT: 301-743-7613;
dnr2.maryland.gov

OPERATED BY: Maryland Department
of Natural Resources

OPEN: Late March–late October

SITES: 15, plus 6 camper cabins

EACH SITE: Picnic table, lantern post,
fire ring

ASSIGNMENT: At headquarters office;
you must check with a ranger prior to
setting up in any of the sites.

REGISTRATION: Recommended
between Memorial and Labor Day;
888-432-CAMP (2267) or
reservations.dnr.state.md.us

FACILITIES: Bathhouse, boat
launch and rental, dumping station,
concessions, marina, picnic shelters,
playground

PARKING: On-site gravel driveway
or the nearest marked parking lot;
2 vehicles/site

FEE: $27.49 plus service charge/night;
additional day-use service charge
$3–$5; boat ramp service charge $10;
out-of-state residents add $2

RESTRICTIONS

▓ **Pets:** Allowed

▓ **Quiet Hours:** 10 p.m.–7 a.m.

▓ **Visitors:** Maximum 6 people/site

▓ **Fires:** In fire rings

▓ **Alcohol:** Permitted only inside
cabins and at shelters with valid
permit, as applicable

▓ **Stay Limit:** 2 weeks; can return after
1 week away

▓ **Other:** Check-in by 8:30 p.m.;
checkout or renew by noon

Visiting Smallwood State Park will give you the distinct feeling that this is a family getaway. The recycled-tire playground plays a large part in that. A nice touch: Most of the playground's equipment is wheelchair accessible. In addition to the restored retreat house, an 18th-century tidewater plantation and 19th-century tobacco barn are also on the grounds, and interpretive guides help visitors know what life was like back then. Craft demonstrations and military exhibitions are held throughout the year. All of these facts mean that bringing kids along is a great idea.

As stated, all campsites are electric. Additionally, none is terribly far from the next, but each is well shaded under mature hardwoods. Some, by virtue of their large size, can offer at least a modicum of privacy. Sites 12, 2, 3, and 1 are the largest, in that order. Because sites are first come, first served, tent campers can have these large sites if they are available. Sites 3–7 (4–6 especially) are farthest from the potential activity of the dump station, playground, and footbridge to the marina.

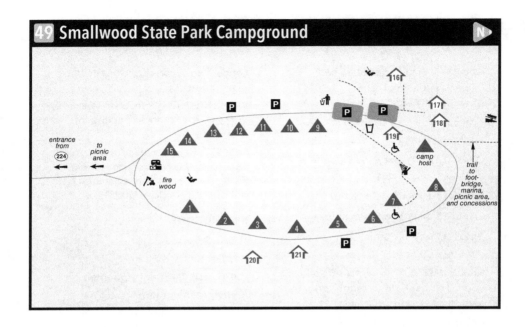

:: Getting There

Take I-495 to Exit 3A, and head south on MD 210. In 17.4 miles, turn left on MD 225, and go 1.6 miles. Turn right on MD 224, and go 3.8 miles. Turn right into the park.

GPS COORDINATES N38°33'23" W77°11'7"

Tuckahoe State Park

There's something about paddling around trees teeming with herons, ospreys, and bald eagles that feels absolutely primeval.

Tuckahoe State Park contains some indispensable American history. The country's most famous abolitionist, Frederick Douglass, was born along Tuckahoe Creek, and the area also served as part of Harriet Tubman's Underground Railroad. Long before the era of American slavery, the Nanticoke Indians, who appreciated the bounty offered by the creek and surrounding marshland forestlands, inhabited Tuckahoe. Today, the area's natural beauty serves as a stark contrast to its difficult past.

The creek, which serves as the dividing line between Queen Anne's and Caroline counties, bisects the park's 3,800 acres and heads eventually to the Choptank River. Tuckahoe Creek also flows into and out of 60-acre Lake Tuckahoe. The park's waterways and forests mean that an almost endless array of recreational opportunities awaits the visitor. Within the park's acreage also lies 500-acre Adkins Arboretum, crisscrossed by 3 miles of hiking trails; in all, the park contains some 20 miles of trail, including for flatwater canoeing. And for kids, there's a nice recycled-tire playground.

Personally, I think the lake's 40 acres of flooded forestland is the most unique attraction. While the rest of the lake is open water and allows for great fishing, there's something about paddling around trees teeming with herons, ospreys, and bald eagles that feels absolutely primeval. Don't worry if you didn't bring a canoe; the park provides rentals (and rents bikes too). Don't worry about noise, either: Gasoline motors are prohibited. For a great experience, explore the park's great water trails and then beach to walk more trails throughout the forest.

Another attraction to Tuckahoe is its isolated feel. A perfect jewel of typical Maryland Eastern Shore scenery, it has so far been spared the rampant development that threatens so much of the Eastern Shore. In fact, you'll be forgiven if upon first visit you think you've taken a

:: Ratings

BEAUTY: ★ ★ ★ ★
PRIVACY: ★ ★ ★ ★
SPACIOUSNESS: ★ ★ ★
QUIET: ★ ★ ★ ★
SECURITY: ★ ★ ★ ★ ★
CLEANLINESS: ★ ★ ★ ★ ★

:: Key Information

ADDRESS: Tuckahoe State Park
13070 Crouse Mill Road
Queen Anne, MD 21657

CONTACT: 410-820-1668;
dnr2.maryland.gov

OPERATED BY: Maryland Department
of Natural Resources

OPEN: Third week of Mar.-Dec.

SITES: 54 (including 6 camper cabins)

EACH SITE: Camping pad, picnic
table, fire ring

ASSIGNMENT: Reservations recommend for weekends

REGISTRATION: 888-432-CAMP
(2267) or **reservations.dnr.state.md.us**

FACILITIES: Bathhouse, playground,
picnic pavilions, arboretum, boat
launch, bike and boat rental

PARKING: In designated spots

FEE: $21.49 plus service charge/night;
$27.49 plus service charge/night
electric

RESTRICTIONS

▪ **Pets:** Allowed on leash

▪ **Quiet Hours:** 11 p.m.-7 a.m.

▪ **Visitors:** Register at camp entrance.

▪ **Fires:** In fire rings

▪ **Alcohol:** Permitted only inside
cabins and at shelters with valid
permit, as applicable

▪ **Stay Limit:** 2 weeks

▪ **Other:** Summertime here means
mosquitoes; be prepared.

wrong turn and are heading to nowhere, with no infrastructure.

As for the camping, there are two loops; the electric one sits closer to the lake, while the nonelectric loop sits just north. The electric loop has 35 sites (1–35) and four cabins. As a general rule, the inner sites on the left side of the inner road tend to sit on slightly higher ground—a consideration if the forecast calls for heavy rain. Three sites in the electric loop (4, 6, and 7) are wheelchair accessible. If tent camping, you'll want to choose the nonelectric loop (sites

36–56), which is smaller, presents easier access to the canoe launch for Tuckahoe Creek, and has a bathhouse in the middle. This loop also offers three tent-only sites (49, 51, and 53), each with a decent buffer of trees. Sites 46–53 are nearest the canoe launch and overflow parking. Otherwise, little distinguishes these sites; they are all generally the same size and sit within a nice copse with sufficient buffer. In short, you really can't go wrong with any of them. This is a lovely place to camp, and it consistently delivers a pleasant experience.

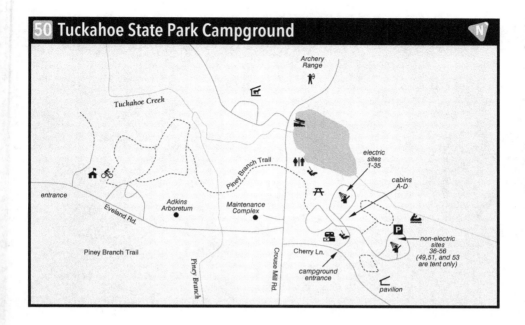

:: Getting There

From Annapolis, head east on US 50/US 301 approximately 30 miles, and take the US 50 E exit toward Ocean City. Continue on US 50 another 6.7 miles, and turn left on MD 404. In 7 miles turn left on MD 480. Take the immediate next left on Eveland Road, and follow it 3.1 miles to Crouse Mill Road; from there, follow the park signs.

GPS COORDINATES N38°58'0" W75°56'34"

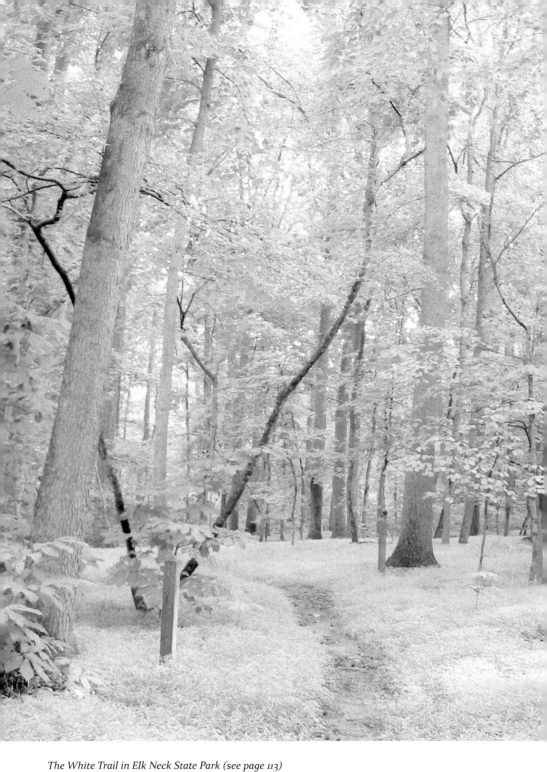

The White Trail in Elk Neck State Park (see page 113)

APPENDIX A

● ●

Camping Equipment Checklist

Except for the large and bulky items on this list, I keep a plastic storage container full of the essentials for car camping so they're ready to go when I am. I make a last-minute check of the inventory, resupply anything that's low or missing, and away I go.

COOKING UTENSILS
Aluminum foil
Bottle opener
Bottles of salt, pepper, spices, sugar, cooking oil, and maple syrup in waterproof, spill-proof containers
Can opener
Corkscrew
Cups, plastic or tin
Dish soap (biodegradable), sponge, and towel
Flatware
Food of your choice
Frying pan
Fuel for stove
Matches in waterproof container
Plates
Pocketknife
Pot with lid
Spatula
Stove
Wooden spoon

FIRST AID KIT
Antibiotic cream
Band-Aids
Diphenhydramine (Benadryl)
Gauze pads
Ibuprofen or aspirin
Insect repellent
Lip balm
Moleskin
Snakebite kit
Sunscreen
Tape, waterproof adhesive

SLEEPING GEAR
Pillow
Sleeping bag
Sleeping pad, inflatable or insulated
Tent with ground tarp and rainfly

MISCELLANEOUS
Bath soap (biodegradable), washcloth, and towel
Camp chair
Candles
Cooler
Deck of cards
Duct tape
Fire starter
Flashlight or headlamp with fresh batteries
Foul-weather clothing
Paper towels
Plastic zip-top bags
Sunglasses
Toilet paper
Water bottle
Wool or fleece blanket

Optional:
Barbecue grill
Binoculars
Field guides on bird, plant, and wildlife identification
Fishing rod and tackle
Hatchet
Kayak and related paddling gear
Lantern
Maps (road, topographic, trails, and so on)
Mountain bike and related riding gear

APPENDIX B

● ●

Sources of Information

**MARYLAND DEPARTMENT OF
NATURAL RESOURCES**
Tawes State Office Building
580 Taylor Ave.
Annapolis, MD 21401
877-620-8DNR or 410-260-8DNR
TTY users call via the MD Relay 711
dnr2.maryland.gov

**MARYLAND-NATIONAL CAPITAL
PARKS AND PLANNING
COMMISSION**
6600 Kenilworth Ave.
Riverdale, MD 20737
301-699-2255
mncppc.org

**MONTGOMERY COUNTY
DEPARTMENT OF PARKS**
9500 Brunett Ave.
Silver Spring, MD 20901
301-495-2595
montgomeryparks.org

NATIONAL PARK SERVICE
1849 C St. NW
Washington, D.C. 20240
202-208-6843
nps.gov

**U.S. ARMY CORPS OF ENGINEERS,
PITTSBURGH DISTRICT**
2200 William S. Moorhead Federal
 Building
1000 Liberty Ave.
Pittsburgh, PA 15222-4186
412-395-7100
www.lrp.usace.army.mil

INDEX

● ●

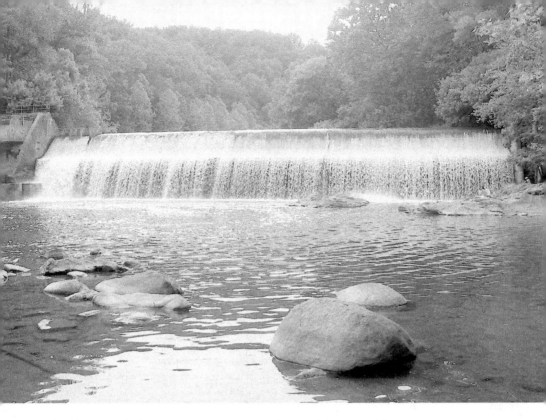

Bloede's Dam in the Hilton area of Patapsco Valley State Park (see page 126)

ABOUT THE AUTHOR

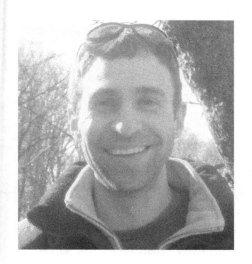

Evan Balkan coordinates the English Department and teaches creative writing at the Community College of Baltimore County. His fiction and nonfiction, mostly in the areas of travel and outdoor recreation, have been published throughout the United States as well as in Canada, England, and Australia. A graduate of Towson, George Mason, and Johns Hopkins Universities, he is also the author of *60 Hikes within 60 Miles: Baltimore; Vanished! Explorers Forever Lost;* and *Shipwrecked! Deadly Adventures and Disasters at Sea* (Menasha Ridge Press), as well as *Walking Baltimore* (Wilderness Press) and *Lope de Aguirre: Revolutionary of the Americas* (University of New Mexico Press). He lives in Towson, Maryland.

DEAR CUSTOMERS AND FRIENDS,

SUPPORTING YOUR INTEREST IN OUTDOOR ADVENTURE, travel, and an active lifestyle is central to our operations, from the authors we choose to the locations we detail to the way we design our books. Menasha Ridge Press was incorporated in 1982 by a group of veteran outdoorsmen and professional outfitters. For many years now, we've specialized in creating books that benefit the outdoors enthusiast.

Almost immediately, Menasha Ridge Press earned a reputation for revolutionizing outdoors- and travel-guidebook publishing. For such activities as canoeing, kayaking, hiking, backpacking, and mountain biking, we established new standards of quality that transformed the whole genre, resulting in outdoor-recreation guides of great sophistication and solid content. Menasha Ridge Press continues to be outdoor publishing's greatest innovator.

The folks at Menasha Ridge Press are as at home on a whitewater river or mountain trail as they are editing a manuscript. The books we build for you are the best they can be, because we're responding to your needs. Plus, we use and depend on them ourselves.

We look forward to seeing you on the river or the trail. If you'd like to contact us directly, visit us at menasharidge.com. We thank you for your interest in our books and the natural world around us all.

SAFE TRAVELS,

Bob Sehlinger

BOB SEHLINGER
PUBLISHER